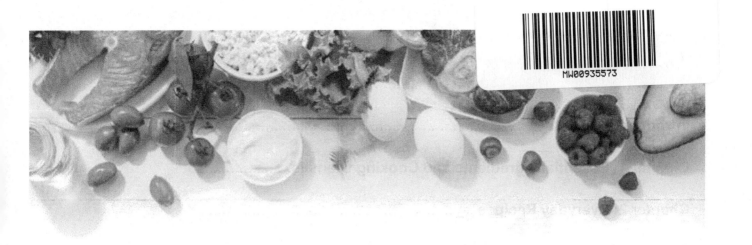

Low-Carb

High-Protein Cookbook

For Beginners

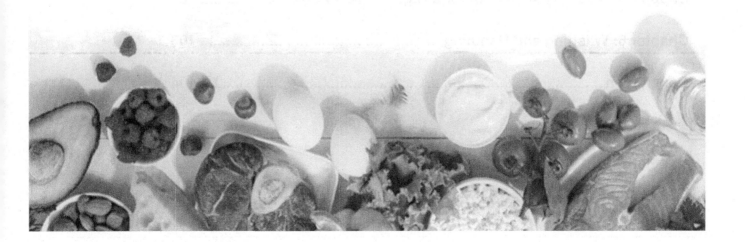

Table of Content

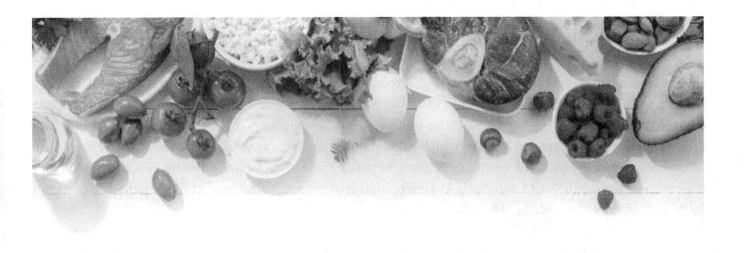

Copyright © by [Feya Adler]

Disclaimer

The information provided in the «Low-carb High-Protein Cookbook for Beginners: 300 Plus Mouthwatering Recipes for Optimal Health, Nurturing the Mind, and Building Muscles, and a 28-day Meal Plan for Weight Management» is for informational purposes only. It is important to note that this guide is not intended as medical or health advice. It should not be used to diagnose, treat, or cure any medical condition or disease. For any such concerns, it is always best to consult with a qualified healthcare professional.

It is important to reiterate that the author and publisher of this guide are not medical professionals. The advice provided here is not intended to replace medical advice. The strategies, tips, and suggestions contained in this guide are not guaranteed to produce specific results and may vary depending on individual circumstances. Therefore, it is strongly advised to consult with a healthcare professional before making any dietary changes or starting any new health regimen.

The author and publisher disclaim any liability directly or indirectly for using the material provided in this guide. By reading this material, you agree that the author and publisher are not responsible for the success or failure of your dietary decisions related to any information presented here.

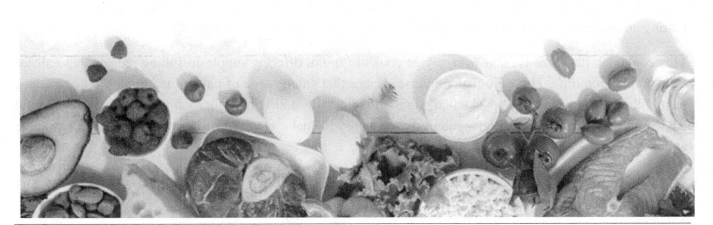

A Personal Note from the Author

Here is where you can get the "Low-Carb High-Protein Cookbook for Beginners." It gives me great pleasure to lead you on this exciting path towards a more lively, healthy living as the book's author. This cookbook is a starting point for changing your perspective on food and nutrition, not just a list of recipes.

I developed a strong interest in low-carb, high-protein nutrition a few years ago while looking for long-term solutions to better my personal health. Like many of you, I came across a lot of food fads and contradictory recommendations. Not until I adopted a low-carb, high-protein, and balanced diet did I notice a significant shift in my energy levels, general health, and connection with food.

This cookbook's recipes and advice are the result of years of research, study, and a sincere passion for preparing tasty, nutritious meals. I created this book with novice cooks in mind, making every meal approachable, entertaining, and filling. I think you'll find something here that suits your tastes and way of life, whether you're new to this type of eating or want to expand your culinary skills.

I recognize that altering one's eating habits might be intimidating. Because of this, this book also offers doable tactics and suggestions to keep you focused and facilitate this shift as much as possible. My mission is to give you all the tools you need to succeed, from meal planning and kitchen necessities to staying motivated.

I appreciate you letting me follow along on your health journey. It is my desire that this cookbook encourages you to taste new cuisines, relish the cooking process, and, above all, fuel your body with health-promoting nutrients.

Introduction

Introducing the "Low-Carb High-Protein Cookbook for Beginners," an all-inclusive manual for adopting a wholesome, fulfilling, and long-lasting diet. Whether you're new to low-carb, high-protein eating or looking to improve your strategy, this cookbook has a plethora of knowledge and delicious recipes to support you in reaching your wellness and health objectives.

Low-carb, high-protein diets have become more and more well-liked in recent years due to their ability to help people lose weight, build muscle, and enhance their general health. You can experience sustained energy levels, enhanced metabolic health, and a stronger feeling of fullness and satisfaction after meals by putting an emphasis on nutrient-dense, high-protein, low-carb foods.

This cookbook has been created with novice cooks in mind, offering simple-to-follow recipes that call for little preparation time. There are many diverse recipes that suit a range of palates and dietary requirements, from filling dinners to tasty snacks and robust brunches. In addition to the recipes, you will get helpful advice on how to maintain a high-protein diet, which will make your path to improved health pleasurable and doable.

Together, let's go on this culinary journey and turn your kitchen into a center for wholesome and delectable dishes. Greetings from a fresh chapter of healthful eating!

Chapter 1: Essential Ingredients and Cooking Utensils

Essential Ingredients

Setting yourself up for success with a low-carb, high-protein diet begins with preparing the necessary foods and appliances in your kitchen. This is a list of necessities that will simplify dinner preparation.

ESSENTIAL COMPONENTS PROTEINS:

Lean meats include turkey, lean beef cuts, and chicken breast.
Fish and Seafood: shellfish such as shrimp, tuna, and salmon.
Plant-Based Proteins: lentils, edamame, tofu, and tempeh.
Eggs: A flexible and high-protein staple food.

DAIRY AND ITS SUBSTITUTES:

Greek yogurt is rich in protein and works well in a variety of recipes.
Cheese: Cottage cheese, cheddar, and mozzarella are examples.
Almond milk without sugar, coconut milk, and soy milk are some milk substitutes.

PRODUCE:

Leafy greens: Swiss chard, arugula, kale, and spinach.
Brussels sprouts, cauliflower, and broccoli are examples of cruciferous vegetables.
Additional Low-Carb Vegetables: Asparagus, bell peppers, and zucchini.

GOOD FATS:

Avocados: A fantastic source of fiber and good fats.
Nuts and seeds: Walnuts, flaxseeds, almonds, and chia seeds.
Oils: avocado, coconut, and olive oils.

PANTRY ESSENTIALS:

Herbs and Spices: paprika, cumin, oregano, turmeric, and basil.
Condiments: Hot sauce, vinegar, mustard, and soy sauce (or tamari for a gluten-free alternative).
Almond flour and coconut flour are low-carb flours.

Kitchen Utensils

ESSENTIAL TOOLS:
Two sharp knives - a paring knife and a chef's knife.
Cutting boards: Ideally keep the ones for veggies and meat separate.
Measuring cups and spoons is necessary to ensure recipe accuracy.

KITCHENWARE:

For purees, sauces, and smoothies, use a blender or food processor.
For simple, hands-off cooking, use an Instant Pot or Slow Cooker.
Non-stick Skillets and Pots: Ideal for cooking a variety of dishes and sautéing them.

ESSENTIAL BAKING INGREDIENTS:

Pans and Baking Sheets: For baking and roasting.

Mixing Bowls: Assorted sizes for blending mixtures.

For simple cleanup and non-stick baking, use parchment paper and silicone mats.

These products and utensils will help you cook excellent, high-protein, low-carb meals that will support your health and culinary objectives. Stock your kitchen with them.

Tips for Sustaining a High-Protein Lifestyle

Changing to a low-carb, high-protein diet might be simple if you know what to do. Here are some pointers to help you maintain this way of life and reap its long-term rewards.

ORGANIZE YOUR MEALS

WEEKLY MEAL PLANNING: Set aside time once a week to organize your snacks and meals. This keeps things interesting and guarantees you have everything you need.

Cooking in bulk can help you save time and guarantee that you always have wholesome food options available. Simply make larger portions of meals that can be frozen and reheated.

MAINTAIN HYDRATION

WATER: Try to have eight glasses or more of water per day. Drinking enough water facilitates digestion and prolongs feelings of fullness.

Limit beverages high in sugar: Steer clear of sugar-filled beverages and choose herbal or water instead.

KEEP AN EYE ON YOUR PROTEIN INTAKE: Make Sure Every Meal Has a Good Source of Protein, Healthy Fats, and Low-Carb Vegetables to Maintain Meal Balance.

Use Protein Supplements: If you're active or trying to gain muscle, use protein powders or bars to help you reach your daily protein targets.

PAY ATTENTION TO YOUR BODY: Identify Your Hunger Cues: Eat till you're satisfied and quit when you're not. By doing this, you can avoid overindulging and keep your weight in check.

MODIFY THE PORTIONS: Adjust the quantity of your portions according to your exercise level and dietary requirements.

CONTINUE TO MOVE

FREQUENT EXERCISE: Make sure your regimen includes both strength and cardio activities. A high-protein diet is complemented by physical activity since it promotes overall fitness and muscular building.

REMAIN STEADY: Discover enjoyable hobbies to help you exercise regularly.

SEEK ASSISTANCE: Join Communities: Participate in local gatherings, social media groups, and online forums centered to high-protein, low-carb lifestyles. Motivation and fresh ideas can be obtained by exchanging recipes and experiences.

SPEAK WITH EXPERTS: To make sure your diet satisfies all of your nutritional requirements and supports your overall health objectives, consult a nutritionist or dietitian.

You can sustain a high-protein, low-carb lifestyle that promotes your overall health and well-being by putting these suggestions into practice on a daily basis.

Chapter 2: Everyday Recipes

2.1 Breakfast

Apple Cinnamon Overnight Oats

Time: 5 minutes (plus 1 night)| Difficulty: Easy| Serving 2

1 cup rolled oats
1 cup almond milk
1 apple, diced
2 tablespoons maple syrup
1/2 teaspoon cinnamon
1/4 teaspoon vanilla extract
Chopped nuts for topping (optional)

1. In a bowl or jar, mix rolled oats, almond milk, diced apple, maple syrup, cinnamon, and vanilla extract.
2. Stir until well combined.
3. Cover and refrigerate overnight, or for at least 4 hours, to allow the oats to absorb the liquid and soften.
4. Stir well before serving.
5. Top with chopped nuts, if desired.

Per Serving
Calories: 250|Protein: 6g|Carbs: 45g|Fat: 6g|Fiber: 7g

Vegetable Frittata

Time: 20 minutes| Difficulty: Easy| Serving 2

4 eggs
1/2 cup diced bell peppers
1/2 cup diced zucchini
1/4 cup diced onions
1/4 cup grated cheese
Salt and pepper to taste
Olive oil for cooking

1. Preheat the oven to 350°F (175°C).
2. In a mixing bowl, whisk together eggs, salt, and pepper until well beaten.
3. Heat olive oil in an oven-safe skillet over medium heat.
4. Add diced onions and cook until translucent.
5. Add diced bell peppers and zucchini to the skillet and cook until softened.
6. Pour the beaten eggs over the vegetables in the skillet.
7. Cook for a few minutes until the edges start to set.
8. Sprinkle grated cheese evenly over the top.
9. Transfer the skillet to the preheated oven and bake for 10-12 minutes, until the frittata is set and golden brown on top.
10. Remove from the oven and let it cool slightly before slicing and serving.

Per Serving
Calories: 250|Protein: 16g|Carbs: 8g|Fat: 15g|Fiber: 2g

Lemon Blueberry Quinoa

Time: 10 minutes| Difficulty: Easy| Serving 2

1 cup cooked quinoa
1/2 cup almond milk
1 tablespoon honey or maple syrup
Zest of 1 lemon
1/2 cup fresh blueberries
2 tablespoons sliced almonds
Fresh mint leaves for garnish (optional)

1. In a saucepan, heat almond milk over medium heat until warm.
2. Stir in cooked quinoa, honey or maple syrup, and lemon zest.
3. Cook, stirring occasionally, until the quinoa is heated through.
4. Divide the quinoa mixture between two bowls.
5. Top each bowl with fresh blueberries and sliced almonds.
6. Garnish with fresh mint leaves, if desired.

Per Serving: Calories: 250|Protein: 6g|Carbs: 40g|Fat: 7g|Fiber: 5g

Healthy Breakfast Burrito Bowl

Time: 20 minutes| Difficulty: Moderate| Serving 2

1 cup cooked quinoa
1/2 cup black beans, drained and rinsed
1/2 avocado, sliced
2 large eggs, scrambled
1/4 cup salsa
1/4 cup shredded cheese (optional)
Salt and pepper to taste

1. In a bowl, layer cooked quinoa, black beans, scrambled eggs, sliced avocado, salsa, and shredded cheese (if using).
2. Season with salt and pepper to taste.
3. Serve immediately.

Per serving:
Calories: 380| Protein: 21g| Fat: 17g| Carbs: 36g

Smoked Salmon and Cream Cheese Bagel

Time: 10 minutes| Difficulty: Easy| Serving 2

2 whole-grain bagels, halved and toasted
4 tablespoons cream cheese
4 slices smoked salmon
1/4 cup sliced cucumber
1/4 cup sliced red onion
Fresh dill for garnish

1. Spread cream cheese evenly onto each toasted bagel half.
2. Top with smoked salmon, sliced cucumber, and sliced red onion.
3. Garnish with fresh dill.

Per serving
Calories: 350| Protein: 20g|Carbs: 30g|Fat: 15g|Fiber: 6g

Lemon Blueberry Quinoa Breakfast Bowl

Time: 10 minutes| Difficulty: Easy| Serving 2

1 cup cooked quinoa
1/2 cup almond milk
1 tablespoon honey or maple syrup
Zest of 1 lemon
1/2 cup fresh blueberries
2 tablespoons sliced almonds
Fresh mint leaves for garnish (optional)

1. In a saucepan, heat almond milk over medium heat until warm.
2. Stir in cooked quinoa, honey or maple syrup, and lemon zest.
3. Cook, stirring occasionally, until the quinoa is heated through.
4. Divide the quinoa mixture between two bowls.
5. Top each bowl with fresh blueberries and sliced almonds.
6. Garnish with fresh mint leaves, if desired.

Per Serving
Calories: 250|Protein: 6g|Carbs: 40g|Fat: 7g|Fiber: 5g

Breakfast Stuffed Sweet Potatoes

Time: 45 minutes| Difficulty: Moderate| Serving 2

2 medium sweet potatoes
4 large eggs, scrambled
1/2 cup black beans, drained and rinsed
1/4 cup diced bell peppers
1/4 cup diced onions
1/4 cup shredded cheese (cheddar or Monterey Jack)
Fresh cilantro for garnish
Salt and pepper to taste
Cooking spray

1. Preheat the oven to 400°F (200°C).
2. Wash and scrub the sweet potatoes, then pierce them several times with a fork.
3. Place the sweet potatoes on a baking sheet lined with parchment paper and bake for 40-45 minutes, or until tender.
4. While the sweet potatoes are baking, prepare the scrambled eggs.
5. Heat a non-stick skillet over medium heat and coat with cooking spray.
6. Sautee the diced onions and bell peppers until softened.
7. Add the scrambled eggs to the skillet and cook until set.
8. Once the sweet potatoes are cooked, slice them open lengthwise and fluff the insides with a fork.
9. Divide the scrambled eggs, black beans, and shredded cheese between the two sweet potatoes.
10. Season with salt and pepper to taste.
11. Garnish with fresh cilantro.
12. Serve immediately.

Per serving
Calories: 320| Protein: 18g| Fat: 12g| Carbs: 35g

Vegetable and Quinoa Breakfast Skillet

Time: 25 minutes| Difficulty: Easy| Serving 2

1 tablespoon olive oil
1/2 cup diced bell peppers
1/2 cup diced zucchini
1/4 cup diced onions
1 clove garlic, minced
1 cup cooked quinoa
2 large eggs
Salt and pepper to taste
Fresh parsley for garnish

1. Heat olive oil in a skillet over medium heat.
2. Add the diced onions and garlic to the skillet and cook until softened.
3. Add the diced bell peppers and zucchini to the skillet and sauté until tender.
4. Stir in the cooked quinoa and cook until heated through.
5. Make two wells in the quinoa mixture and crack an egg into each well.
6. Cover the skillet and cook until the eggs are set to your liking (about 3-5 minutes for runny yolks).
7. Season with salt and pepper to taste.
8. Garnish with fresh parsley.
9. Serve immediately.

Per serving
Calories: 290| Protein: 14g| Fat: 12g| Carbs: 30g

Egg and Vegetable Frittata

Time: 20 minutes| Difficulty: Easy| Serving 2

4 eggs
1/2 cup chopped vegetables (such as bell peppers, onions, spinach)
1/4 cup shredded cheese (optional)
Salt and pepper to taste
Olive oil for cooking

1. Preheat the oven to 350°F (175°C).
2. Whisk together eggs, salt, and pepper in a bowl until well beaten.
3. Heat olive oil in an oven-safe skillet over medium heat.
4. Add chopped vegetables to the skillet and cook until softened.
5. Pour the beaten eggs over the vegetables in the skillet, ensuring they are evenly distributed.
6. Cook for 3-4 minutes, until the edges begin to set.
7. Sprinkle shredded cheese over the top (if using).
8. Transfer the skillet to the preheated oven and bake for 10-12 minutes, or until the frittata is set and golden brown on top.
9. Remove from the oven and let it cool slightly before slicing.

Per Serving
Calories: 180|Protein: 12g|Carbs: 8g|Fat: 10g|Fiber: 2g

Spinach and Mushroom Omelette

Time: 15 minutes| Difficulty: Easy| Serving 2

4 eggs
1 cup fresh spinach leaves
1/2 cup sliced mushrooms
1/4 cup shredded cheese (optional)
Salt and pepper to taste
Olive oil for cooking

1. In a bowl, whisk together eggs, salt, and pepper until well beaten.
2. Heat olive oil in a skillet over medium heat.
3. Add sliced mushrooms to the skillet and cook until softened.
4. Add fresh spinach leaves to the skillet and cook until wilted.
5. Pour the beaten eggs over the mushrooms and spinach in the skillet.
6. Cook for 3-4 minutes, until the eggs are set but still moist.
7. Sprinkle shredded cheese over the top (if using).
8. Fold the omelet in half and cook for another minute to melt the cheese

Per serving
Calories: 200|Protein: 14g|Carbs: 5g|Fat: 14g|Fiber: 2g

Quinoa Breakfast Bowl with Sautéed Vegetables

Time: 20 minutes| Difficulty: Easy| Serving 2

1 cup cooked quinoa
1/2 cup diced bell peppers
1/2 cup diced zucchini
1/4 cup diced onions
2 cloves garlic, minced
2 eggs
Salt and pepper to taste
Olive oil for cooking

1. Heat olive oil in a skillet over medium heat.
2. Add diced onions and minced garlic to the skillet and cook until fragrant.
3. Add diced bell peppers and zucchini to the skillet and sauté until softened.
4. Stir in cooked quinoa and continue to cook until heated through.
5. In a separate skillet, cook eggs to your desired doneness (such as sunny-side-up or scrambled).
6. Divide the quinoa and sautéed vegetables between two bowls.
7. Top each bowl with a cooked egg.
8. Season with salt and pepper to taste.

Per serving
Calories: 300|Protein: 12g| Carbs: 30g| Fat: 15g|Fiber: 6g

Avocado Toast with Poached Eggs

Time: 10 minutes| Difficulty: Easy| Serving 2

2 slices whole-grain bread
1 ripe avocado
4 eggs
Fresh herbs for garnish
Red pepper flakes (optional)
Salt and black pepper

1. Toast the slices of whole-grain bread until golden brown.
2. While the bread is toasting, mash the ripe avocado in a small bowl and season with salt, pepper, and red pepper flakes (if using).
3. Poach the eggs in simmering water until the whites are set, but the yolks are still runny.
4. Spread the mashed avocado evenly onto the toasted bread slices.
5. Top each slice with two poached eggs.
6. Garnish with fresh herbs, such as chopped parsley or chives.

Per Serving: Calories: 300|Protein: 12g|Carbs: 20g|Fat: 20g|Fiber: 8g

Mediterranean Breakfast Plate

Time: 15 minutes| Difficulty: Easy| Serving 2

2 large eggs, boiled and sliced
1/2 cup cherry tomatoes, halved
1/4 cucumber, sliced
1/4 cup hummus
2 whole wheat pita bread, toasted
Kalamata olives for garnish
Fresh parsley for garnish

1. Arrange boiled egg slices, cherry tomatoes, cucumber slices, and whole wheat pita bread on a plate.
2. Serve with a dollop of hummus.
3. Garnish with Kalamata olives and fresh parsley.
4. Serve immediately.

Per serving: Calories: 340| Protein: 18g| Fat: 14g| Carbs: 38g

Protein-Packed Breakfast Bowl

Time: 15 minutes| Difficulty: Easy |Serving 2

2 cups cooked quinoa
4 eggs
1 avocado, sliced
1/2 cup cherry tomatoes, halved
1/4 cup crumbled feta cheese
Salt and pepper to taste
Olive oil for cooking

1. In a skillet, cook eggs to your desired doneness (such as scrambled or sunny-side-up).
2. Divide cooked quinoa between two serving bowls.
3. Top each bowl with cooked eggs, sliced avocado, cherry tomatoes, and crumbled feta cheese.
4. Season with salt and pepper to taste.
5. Drizzle with olive oil, if desired.

Per serving: Calories: 400|Protein: 20g| Carbs: 30g|Fat: 25g|Fiber: 8g

Egg and Avocado Breakfast Burrito

Time: 25 minutes| Difficulty: Moderate| Serving 2

4 large eggs
2 whole wheat tortillas
*1 avocado, sliced **and** 1 tablespoon olive oil*
1/2 cup black beans, drained and rinsed
*1/4 cup salsa **and** Salt and pepper to taste*

1. In a bowl, whisk together eggs, salt, and pepper.
2. Heat olive oil in a skillet over medium heat. Pour in the egg mixture and cook, stirring occasionally, until the eggs are scrambled and cooked through.
3. Warm the whole wheat tortillas in the skillet or microwave for a few seconds until they are pliable.
4. Divide the scrambled eggs, sliced avocado, black beans, and salsa between the tortillas.
5. Roll up the tortillas to form burritos, tucking in the sides as you go.
6. Serve immediately, or wrap the burritos in foil for an on-the-go breakfast.

Per serving
Calories: 320| Protein: 15g| Fat: 18g| Carbs: 26

Turkish Menemen (Scrambled Eggs with Vegetables)

Time: 25 minutes| Difficulty: Easy| Serving 2

4 eggs
1 onion, chopped
1 green bell pepper, chopped
2 tomatoes, diced
1/2 tsp. paprika
Salt and pepper to taste
2 tbsp. parsley, chopped
1 tbsp. olive oil

1. Heat olive oil in a skillet and sauté onions and bell pepper until soft.
2. Add tomatoes and paprika, cooking until the mixture is saucy.
3. Scramble eggs into the mixture until cooked.
4. Garnish with parsley before serving.

Per serving
Calories: 240| Protein: 14g| Fat: 17g| Carbs: 10g

Egg and Avocado Breakfast Wrap

Time: 10 minutes| Difficulty: Easy| Serving 2

4 eggs
1 ripe avocado, sliced
2 whole-wheat tortillas
Salt and pepper to taste
Salsa for serving (optional)

1. In a skillet, scramble the eggs until cooked through.
2. Warm the whole-wheat tortillas in the skillet or microwave.
3. Divide scrambled eggs and sliced avocado between the tortillas.
4. Season with salt and pepper to taste.
5. Roll up the tortillas to form wraps.
6. Serve with salsa on the side, if desired

Per serving:
Calories: 300| Protein: 14g| Carbs: 20g| Fat: 18g| Fiber: 6g

2.2 Salad Recipes

Tuna Salad Lettuce

Time: 10 minutes| Difficulty: Easy| Serving 2

1 can tuna, drained
2 tablespoons Greek yogurt
1 tablespoon lemon juice
Salt and pepper, to taste
Lettuce leaves, for wrapping
Tomato slices, for topping

1. In a bowl, mix together tuna, Greek yogurt, lemon juice, salt, and pepper.
2. Spoon tuna salad onto lettuce leaves.
3. Top with tomato slices.
4. Roll up lettuce leaves to form wraps.
5. Serve immediately for a protein-rich and satisfying snack.

Per serving
Calories: 150| Protein: 15g| Carbs: 5g| Fat: 7g| Fiber: 2g

Mediterranean Chickpea Salad

Time: 15 minutes| Difficulty: Easy| Serving 2

1 can (15 ounces) chickpeas, rinsed and drained
1 cup cherry tomatoes, halved
1 cucumber, diced
1/4 cup red onion, thinly sliced
1/4 cup of olives, pitted and halved
2 tablespoons chopped fresh parsley
Juice of 1 lemon
2 tablespoons extra virgin olive oil
Salt and pepper to taste

1. In a large bowl, combine the chickpeas, cherry tomatoes, cucumber, red onion, olives, and chopped parsley.
2. In a small bowl, whisk together the lemon juice, extra virgin olive oil, salt, and pepper to make the dressing.
3. Pour the dressing over the salad ingredients and toss until well combined.

Per serving
Calories: 250| Carbohydrates: 30g| Fats: 10g| Protein: 10g

Grilled Chicken Salad with Mixed Greens

Time: 35 minutes| Difficulty: Easy| Serving 2

2 boneless, skinless chicken breasts (about 6 oz. each)
1 tablespoon olive oil, plus extra for grilling
4 cups mixed greens (such as lettuce, arugula, and spinach)
1 medium cucumber, thinly sliced
1/2 cup cherry tomatoes, halved
1/4 red onion, thinly sliced
1/4 cup crumbled feta cheese
2 tablespoons balsamic vinegar
1 teaspoon honey
1 teaspoon Dijon mustard
1 tablespoon water
Salt and pepper to taste

1. Preheat Grill: Preheat your grill medium-high heat and brush it with a bit of olive oil.
2. Season Chicken: Season the chicken breasts with salt and pepper, then drizzle with 1 tablespoon of olive oil to coat evenly.
3. Grill Chicken: Place the chicken on the grill and cook for about 5-7 minutes on each side, or until fully cooked through and the internal temperature reaches 165°F (74°C). Once cooked, remove from the grill and let it rest for a few minutes. Then, slice thinly.
4. Prepare Salad Dressing: In a small bowl, whisk together balsamic vinegar, honey, Dijon mustard, and water until well combined. Season with a pinch of salt and pepper to taste.
5. Assemble the Salad: In a large bowl, combine mixed greens, cucumber slices, cherry tomatoes, and red onion slices. Drizzle with the prepared dressing and toss gently to coat.
6. Serve: Divide the salad onto plates, top with sliced grilled chicken and crumbled feta cheese. Serve immediately.

Per serving
Calories: 350| Carbs: 12g| Fats: 16g| Protein: 36g

Quinoa and Black Bean Salad

Time: 30 minutes| Difficulty: Easy| Serving 2

1 cup cooked quinoa (cooled)
1 can (15 oz.) black beans, rinsed and drained
1 red bell pepper, diced
1/4 cup fresh cilantro, chopped
2 green onions, sliced
Juice of 1 lime
2 tablespoons olive oil
Salt and pepper to taste

1. In a large bowl, combine the quinoa, black beans, red bell pepper, cilantro, and green onions.
2. In a small bowl, whisk together lime juice, olive oil, salt, and pepper.
3. Pour the dressing over the quinoa mixture and toss to combine.
4. Serve immediately or refrigerate until ready to serve.

Per serving
Calories: 320 | Carbs: 45g| Fats: 9g| Protein: 12g

Shrimp and Quinoa Salad

Time: 35 minutes| Difficulty: Moderate| Serving 2

1/2 cup quinoa, rinsed
1 cup water
200g (about 7 oz.) shrimp, peeled and deveined
1 tablespoon olive oil
1/2 teaspoon paprika
Salt and pepper to taste
1 cup cherry tomatoes, halved
1/2 cucumber, diced
1/4 red onion, finely sliced
1 avocado, diced
1/4 cup chopped fresh cilantro (or parsley, if preferred)
Juice of 1 lime
2 tablespoons extra-virgin olive oil
Mixed greens (optional, for serving)

1. Cook Quinoa: In a medium saucepan, bring 1 cup of water to a boil. Add quinoa and a pinch of salt, reduce heat to low, cover, and simmer for 15 minutes or until all the water is absorbed. Remove from heat and let it sit, covered, for 5 minutes. Fluff with a fork and let cool.
2. Prepare Shrimp: While the quinoa is cooking, season shrimp with 1 tablespoon of olive oil, paprika, salt, and pepper. Heat a pan over medium-high heat and cook the shrimp for 2-3 minutes on each side, or until they turn pink and opaque. Remove from heat and set aside to cool.
3. Assemble Salad: In a large bowl, combine the cooked quinoa, cooled shrimp, cherry tomatoes, cucumber, red onion, and avocado. Add the chopped cilantro (or parsley) and gently mix to combine.
4. Dressing: In a small bowl, whisk together lime juice and 2 tablespoons of extra-virgin olive oil. Season with salt and pepper to taste. Pour the dressing over the salad and toss to evenly coat.
5. Serve: Serve the salad on a bed of mixed greens, if using, for an additional nutrient boost.

Per serving : Calories: Approx. 400|Carbohydrates: 33g| Fats: 22g| Protein: 24g

Black Bean and Corn Salad with Avocado

Time: 15 minutes| Difficulty: Easy| Serving 2

1 can (15 ounces) black beans, rinsed and drained
1 cup corn kernels (fresh, canned, or frozen)
1 avocado, diced
1/2 red bell pepper, diced
1/4 cup red onion, finely chopped
1/4 cup fresh cilantro, chopped
Juice of 1 lime
2 tablespoons extra virgin olive oil
1 teaspoon ground cumin
Salt and pepper to taste

1. Prepare the Salad Ingredients: In a large mixing bowl, combine the black beans, corn kernels, diced avocado, diced red bell pepper, chopped red onion, and chopped cilantro.
2. Make the Dressing: In a small bowl, whisk together the lime juice, extra virgin olive oil, ground cumin, salt, and pepper until well combined.
3. Combine Salad and Dressing: Pour the dressing over the salad ingredients in the mixing bowl. Gently toss until everything is evenly coated with the dressing.
4. Adjust Seasoning: Taste the salad and adjust the seasoning with additional salt and pepper if needed.
5. Serve: Transfer the black bean and corn salad to serving bowls or plates. Enjoy immediately as a light and refreshing meal or side dish.

Per serving: Calories: 250| Carbs: 27g| Fats: 13g| Protein: 6g

Greek Salad with Grilled Chicken

Time: 35 minutes| Difficulty: Easy| Serving 2

2 boneless, skinless chicken breasts (about 6 ounces each)
1 tablespoon olive oil
1 teaspoon dried oregano
Salt and pepper to taste
4 cups mixed salad greens (like romaine, arugula, and spinach)
1 large tomato, chopped
1 cucumber, sliced
1/2 red onion, thinly sliced
1/2 cup olives, pitted
1/2 cup crumbled feta cheese

Ingredients for the Dressing*:*
3 tablespoons extra virgin olive oil
1 tablespoon red wine vinegar
1 teaspoon Dijon mustard
1 garlic clove, minced
Salt and pepper to taste

1. Prep the Chicken: Preheat your grill or grill pan over medium heat. Season the chicken breasts with olive oil, dried oregano, salt, and pepper.
2. Grill the Chicken: Place the chicken on the grill and cook for about 5 minutes per side, or until fully cooked through and the internal temperature reaches 165°F (74°C). Once cooked, let it rest for a few minutes before slicing thinly.
3. Mix the Dressing: In a small bowl, whisk together the extra virgin olive oil, red wine vinegar, Dijon mustard, minced garlic, salt, and pepper. Set aside.
4. Assemble the Salad: In a large salad bowl, combine the mixed greens, chopped tomato, sliced cucumber, red onion, olives, and crumbled feta cheese. Toss to mix.
5. Add Chicken and Dressing: Add the sliced grilled chicken to the salad and drizzle with the prepared dressing. Toss lightly to ensure everything is well coated.
6. Serve: Divide the salad between two plates and serve immediately.

Per serving
Calories: 550| Carbohydrates: 12g| Fats: 36g| Protein: 44g

Warm Beetroot and Goat Cheese Salad

Time: 25 minutes| Difficulty: Easy| Serving 2

2 medium beetroots, peeled and diced
50g goat cheese, crumbled
2 cups arugula
1 tbsp olive oil
2 tbsp balsamic glaze and Salt and pepper to taste
1. Roast beetroot in a preheated oven at 400°F for 20 minutes.
2. Toss warm beetroot with arugula and goat cheese.
3. Drizzle with olive oil and balsamic glaze, season with salt and pepper, and serve.

Per serving
Calories: 180| Protein: 6g| Fat: 10g| Carbs: 18g

Asian Cabbage Salad with Grilled Chicken

Time: 25 minutes| Difficulty: Moderate| Serving 2

2 boneless, skinless chicken breasts
4 cups shredded cabbage (green or Napa)
1 cup shredded carrots
1/4 cup sliced green onions
1/4 cup chopped cilantro
1/4 cup chopped peanuts
2 tablespoons sesame seeds
2 tablespoons rice vinegar
1 tablespoon soy sauce
1 tablespoon honey
1 teaspoon grated ginger
1 garlic clove, minced **and** *Salt and pepper to taste*

1. Season the chicken breasts with salt and pepper, then grill until cooked through. Let them rest for a few minutes before slicing thinly.
2. In a large bowl, combine the shredded cabbage, shredded carrots, sliced green onions, chopped cilantro, chopped peanuts, and sesame seeds.
3. In a small bowl, whisk together the rice vinegar, soy sauce, honey, grated ginger, minced garlic, salt, and pepper to make the dressing.
4. Pour the dressing over the salad ingredients and toss until well combined.
5. Serve the salad topped with sliced grilled chicken.

Per Serving
Calories: 350| Carbohydrates: 20g| Fats: 15g| Protein: 30g

Warm Broccoli and Chicken Salad

Time: 20 minutes| Difficulty: Easy| Serving 2

2 cups broccoli florets
1 cooked chicken breast, sliced
- 1/4 cup sliced almonds
- 2 tbsp. dried cranberries
- 1 tbsp. olive oil
- 1 tbsp. lemon juice
- Salt and pepper to taste

1. Steam broccoli until tender-crisp, about 5 minutes.
2. In a skillet, toast almonds until lightly golden.
3. Toss warm broccoli, chicken, almonds, and cranberries together.
4. Drizzle with olive oil and lemon juice, season with salt and pepper, and serve warm.

Per serving
Calories: 280| Protein: 25g| Fat: 14g| Carbs: 16g

Warm Chicken and Avocado Salad

Time: 20 minutes| Difficulty: Easy| Serving 2

2 cooked chicken breasts, sliced
1 ripe avocado, sliced
2 cups mixed salad greens
1/2 cucumber, sliced
1 tbsp. olive oil
2 tbsp. lime juice and Salt and pepper to taste
1. In a bowl, combine chicken, avocado, and cucumber.
2. Over medium heat, briefly warm the mixture in a skillet just to take the chill off.
3. Remove from heat and toss with salad greens.
4. Dress with olive oil, lime juice, salt, and pepper, and serve immediately.

Per serving: Calories: 290| Protein: 25g| Fat: 17g| Carbs: 8g

Warm Lentil and Turkey Salad

Time: 30 minutes| Difficulty: Medium| Serving 2

1 cup cooked lentils
1/2 lb. cooked turkey breast, shredded
1 red bell pepper, diced
1/2 red onion, thinly sliced
1 tbsp. olive oil
2 tbsp. cider vinegar
1 tsp. Dijon mustard
Salt and pepper to taste
1. In a skillet, heat olive oil over medium heat.
2. Add bell pepper and onion, sauté until soft.
3. Stir in lentils and turkey, cook until warm.
4. Whisk together cider vinegar, mustard, salt, and pepper.
5. Toss the warm salad with the dressing and serve.

Per serving: Calories: 260| Protein: 28g| Fat: 8g| Carbs: 20g

Warm Shrimp and Avocado Salad

Time: 20 minutes| Difficulty: Easy| Serving 2

1 lb. cooked shrimp, peeled and deveined
1 avocado, diced
2 cups mixed salad greens
1/4 cup sliced cherry tomatoes
2 tbsp. chopped fresh cilantro
1 tbsp. lime juice
1 tbsp. olive oil and Salt and pepper to taste
1. In a large bowl, combine cooked shrimp, avocado, salad greens, and cherry tomatoes.
2. Drizzle with olive oil and lime juice, season with salt and pepper, and toss to combine.
3. Sprinkle with chopped cilantro, and serve warm.

Per serving:
Calories: 240| Protein: 20g| Fat: 14g| Carbs: 10g

Warm Potato and Green Bean Salad

Time: 25 minutes| Difficulty: Easy| Serving 2

2 cups small potatoes, halved
1 cup green beans, trimmed
2 tbsp. olive oil
2 tbsp. red wine vinegar
1 tsp. Dijon mustard **and** *Salt and pepper to taste*
1. Boil potatoes until tender; add green beans in the last 4 minutes of cooking.
2. Drain and while still warm, toss with olive oil, vinegar, mustard, salt, and pepper.
3. Serve warm.

Per serving:
Calories: 220| Protein: 4g| Fat: 10g| Carbs: 30g

Warm Chicken and Couscous Salad

Time: 30 minutes| Difficulty: Easy| Serving 2

2 boneless, skinless chicken breasts
1 cup cooked couscous
1/4 cup sliced almonds and 1/4 cup dried cranberries
2 tbsp. chopped fresh parsley
1 tbsp. lemon juice
1 tbsp. olive oil and Salt and pepper to taste
1. Season chicken breasts with salt and pepper.
2. Grill or pan-fry chicken until cooked through. Slice into strips.
3. In a large bowl, combine cooked couscous, sliced chicken, almonds, cranberries, and parsley.
4. Drizzle with olive oil and lemon juice, toss to combine, and serve warm.

Per serving
Calories: 300| Protein: 25g| Fat: 12g| Carbs: 23g

Warm Quinoa and Roasted Vegetable Salad

Time: 30 minutes| Difficulty: Easy| Serving 2

1 cup cooked quinoa
2 cups mixed roasted vegetables (e.g., bell peppers, eggplant, squash)
1/4 cup crumbled feta cheese
2 tbsp. chopped fresh parsley
1 tbsp. balsamic vinegar
1 tbsp. olive oil
Salt and pepper to taste
1. In a bowl, combine cooked quinoa and roasted vegetables.
2. Drizzle with olive oil and balsamic vinegar, season with salt and pepper, and toss to combine.
3. Sprinkle with crumbled feta cheese and chopped parsley, and serve warm.

Per serving
Calories: 260| Protein: 8g| Fat: 10g| Carbs: 35g

Warm Spinach and Bacon Salad

Time: 25 minutes| Difficulty: Easy| Serving 2

4 cups baby spinach
4 slices bacon, cooked and crumbled
1/4 cup sliced red onion
1/4 cup sliced mushrooms
2 tablespoons olive oil
2 tablespoons apple cider vinegar
1 teaspoon Dijon mustard
Salt and pepper to taste

1. In a skillet, cook bacon until crispy. Remove from skillet and crumble.
2. In the same skillet, add sliced mushrooms and red onion. Sauté until softened.
3. In a small bowl, whisk together olive oil, apple cider vinegar, Dijon mustard, salt, and pepper to make the dressing.
4. In a large bowl, combine baby spinach, crumbled bacon, sautéed mushrooms, and red onion.
5. Drizzle dressing over the salad and toss gently to combine.

Per serving
Calories: 280 Protein: 8g Fat: 22g Carbs: 8g

Warm Potato and Bacon Salad

Time: 40 minutes| Difficulty: Moderate| Serving 2

2 cups baby potatoes, halved
4 slices bacon, cooked and crumbled
1/4 cup diced red onion
2 tablespoons chopped parsley
2 tablespoons olive oil
1 tablespoon white wine vinegar
1 teaspoon Dijon mustard
Salt and pepper to taste

1. Boil baby potatoes in salted water until fork-tender. Drain and set aside.
2. In a skillet, heat olive oil over medium heat. Add diced red onion and sauté until softened.
3. In a small bowl, whisk together white wine vinegar, Dijon mustard, salt, and pepper to make the dressing.
4. In a large bowl, combine cooked baby potatoes, crumbled bacon, sautéed red onion, chopped parsley, and dressing. Toss gently to combine.

Per serving
Calories: 300 Protein: 8g Fat: 18g Carbs: 25g

Warm Lentil and Bacon Salad

Time: 40 minutes| Difficulty: Moderate| Serving 2

1 cup green lentils
4 slices bacon, cooked and crumbled
1/4 cup diced red onion
1/4 cup diced bell pepper
2 tablespoons olive oil
2 tablespoons red wine vinegar
1 teaspoon honey
Salt and pepper to taste

1. Cook lentils according to package instructions.
2. In a skillet, heat olive oil over medium heat. Add diced red onion and bell pepper. Sauté until softened.
3. In a small bowl, whisk together red wine vinegar, honey, salt, and pepper to make the dressing.
4. In a large bowl, combine cooked lentils, crumbled bacon, sautéed red onion, and bell pepper. Drizzle dressing over the salad and toss gently to combine.

Per serving: Calories: 320 Protein: 18g Fat: 12g Carbs: 35g

Warm Lentil and Roasted Vegetable Salad

Time: 40 minutes| Difficulty: Moderate| Serving 2

1 cup dried green lentils
2 cups mixed vegetables (carrots, red onion, bell peppers)
2 tablespoons olive oil
1 teaspoon cumin
Salt and pepper to taste
2 cups arugula
1/4 cup crumbled goat cheese
2 tablespoons lemon juice

1. Cook lentils according to package instructions.
2. Toss mixed vegetables with olive oil, cumin, salt, and pepper. Roast in the oven at 400°F (200°C) for 25 minutes.
3. In a large bowl, combine cooked lentils, roasted vegetables, arugula, and crumbled goat cheese.
4. Drizzle lemon juice over the salad and toss gently to combine.

Per serving: Calories: 320 Protein: 18g Fat: 10g Carbs: 40g

Warm Black Bean and Corn Salad

Time: 20 minutes| Difficulty: Easy| Serving 2

1 can (15 oz.) black beans, rinsed and drained
1 cup frozen corn, thawed
1/2 red bell pepper, diced
1/4 cup chopped red onion
2 tbsp. chopped fresh cilantro
1 tbsp. lime juice
1 tbsp. olive oil
1/2 tsp. ground cumin and Salt and pepper to taste

1. In a skillet, heat olive oil over medium heat. Add corn and cook until lightly browned.
2. In a large bowl, combine black beans, corn, bell pepper, onion, and cilantro.
3. In a small bowl, whisk together lime juice, olive oil, cumin, salt, and pepper.
4. Drizzle the dressing over the salad, toss to combine, and serve warm.

Per serving: Calories: 180| Protein: 7g| Fat: 5g| Carbs: 28g

Chicken and Rice Soup

Time: 40 minutes| Difficulty: Moderate| Serving 2

4 cups chicken broth
2 boneless, skinless chicken breasts
1/2 cup uncooked rice
1 onion, chopped
2 carrots, sliced
2 celery stalks, sliced
1 garlic clove, minced
1 tablespoon olive oil **and** *Salt and pepper to taste*

1. In a large pot, heat olive oil over medium heat. Add chopped onion and minced garlic, cook until fragrant.
2. Add sliced carrots and celery to the pot and cook for a few minutes.
3. Pour in chicken broth and bring to a boil. Add chicken breasts and rice to the pot.
4. Reduce heat and simmer for 20-25 minutes, or until chicken is cooked through and rice is tender.
5. Remove chicken breasts from the pot, shred with forks, and return to the pot.
6. Season with salt and pepper to taste.

Per Serving
Calories 250|Carbohydrates: 20g| Fats: 6g| Protein: 25g

Lentil Soup

Time: 45 minutes| Difficulty: Easy| Serving 2

1 cup dried lentils, rinsed and drained
4 cups vegetable broth
1 onion, chopped
2 carrots, sliced
2 celery stalks, sliced
2 garlic cloves, minced
1 teaspoon ground cumin
1 teaspoon ground coriander
1 tablespoon olive oil **and** *Salt and pepper to taste*

1. Heat olive oil in a large pot over medium heat. Add chopped onion and minced garlic, cook until softened.
2. Add sliced carrots and celery to the pot and cook for a few minutes.
3. Stir in dried lentils, ground cumin, and ground coriander. Cook for another minute.
4. Pour in vegetable broth and bring to a boil. Reduce heat and simmer for 30-35 minutes, or until lentils are tender.
5. Season with salt and pepper to taste.

Per Serving
Calories: 200|Carbohydrates: 30g| Fats: 3g| Protein: 12g

Minestrone Soup

Time: 40 minutes| Difficulty: Moderate| Serving 2

4 cups vegetable broth
1 can (15 ounces) diced tomatoes
1 onion, chopped
2 carrots, sliced
2 celery stalks, sliced
1 zucchini, diced
1 cup cooked pasta (such as small shells or elbow macaroni)
1/2 cup cooked kidney beans
1/4 cup chopped fresh parsley
1 tablespoon olive oil
Salt and pepper to taste

1. Heat olive oil in a large pot over medium heat. Add chopped onion and cook until translucent.
2. Add sliced carrots, sliced celery, and diced zucchini to the pot. Cook for a few minutes until slightly softened.
3. Pour in vegetable broth and diced tomatoes with their juices. Bring to a boil, then reduce heat and simmer for 20-25 minutes.
4. Stir in cooked pasta, cooked kidney beans, and chopped fresh parsley. Cook for an additional 5 minutes.

Per serving
Calories: 220| Carbs: 35g| Fats: 5g| Protein: 8g

Broccoli Cheddar Soup

Time: 35 minutes| Difficulty: Moderate| Serving 2

4 cups vegetable broth
2 cups chopped broccoli florets
1 onion, chopped
2 garlic cloves, minced
1 cup shredded cheddar cheese
1/2 cup milk (or dairy-free alternative)
2 tablespoons olive oil
Salt and pepper to taste

1. Heat olive oil in a large pot over medium heat. Add chopped onion and minced garlic, cook until softened.
2. Add chopped broccoli florets to the pot. Pour in vegetable broth and bring to a boil. Reduce heat and simmer for 15-20 minutes, or until broccoli is tender.
3. Use an immersion blender to puree the soup until smooth.
4. Stir in shredded cheddar cheese and milk, continue to cook until cheese is melted and soup is heated through.
5. Season with salt and pepper to taste.

Per serving
Calories: 250| Carbs: 15g| Fats: 15g| Protein: 10g

Mushroom Barley Soup

Time: 50 minutes| Difficulty: Moderate| Serving 2

4 cups vegetable broth
1 cup pearl barley
8 ounces mushrooms, sliced
1 onion, chopped
2 garlic cloves, minced
1/4 cup chopped fresh dill
2 tablespoons olive oil
Salt and pepper to taste

1. Heat olive oil in a large pot over medium heat. Add chopped onion and minced garlic, cook until softened.
2. Add sliced mushrooms to the pot and cook until tender.
3. Stir in pearl barley and vegetable broth. Bring to a boil, then reduce heat and simmer for 30-35 minutes, or until barley is tender.
4. Stir in chopped fresh dill.
5. Season with salt and pepper to taste.
6. Serve hot.

Per serving
Calories: 200| Carbs: 30g| Fats: 5g| Protein: 7g

Black Bean Soup

Time: 45 minutes| Difficulty: Easy| Serving 2

4 cups vegetable broth
2 cans (15 ounces each) black beans, rinsed and drained
1 onion, chopped
2 garlic cloves, minced
1 bell pepper, chopped
1 jalapeno pepper, seeded and chopped (optional)
1 teaspoon ground cumin
1 teaspoon chili powder
2 tablespoons olive oil
Salt and pepper to taste

1. Heat olive oil in a large pot over medium heat. Add chopped onion and minced garlic, cook until softened.
2. Add chopped bell pepper and jalapeno pepper to the pot. Cook for a few minutes until softened.
3. Stir in ground cumin and chili powder.
4. Pour in vegetable broth and add black beans to the pot. Bring to a boil, then reduce heat and simmer for 20-25 minutes.
5. Use an immersion blender to puree some of the soup, leaving some beans whole for texture.

Per serving
Calories: 220| Carbs: 30g| Fats: 5g| Protein: 10g

Spinach and White Bean Soup

Time: 40 minutes| Difficulty: Easy| Serving 2

4 cups vegetable broth
1 can (15 ounces) white beans, rinsed and drained
2 cups fresh spinach leaves
1 onion, chopped
2 garlic cloves, minced
1 teaspoon dried thyme
1 tablespoon olive oil
Salt and pepper to taste

1. Heat olive oil in a large pot over medium heat. Add chopped onion and minced garlic, cook until softened.
2. Stir in dried thyme.
3. Pour in vegetable broth and add white beans to the pot. Bring to a boil, then reduce heat and simmer for 15-20 minutes.
4. Add fresh spinach leaves to the pot and cook until wilted.
5. Season with salt and pepper to taste.

Per serving
Calories: 180| Carbs: 25g| Fats: 3g| Protein: 10g

Chicken Noodle Soup

Time: 40 minutes| Difficulty: Easy| Serving 2

4 cups chicken broth
2 boneless, skinless chicken breasts
1 cup uncooked egg noodles
1 carrot, sliced
1 celery stalk, sliced
1/2 onion, chopped
2 garlic cloves, minced
1 tablespoon olive oil
Salt and pepper to taste

1. Heat olive oil in a large pot over medium heat. Add chopped onion and minced garlic, cook until softened.
2. Add sliced carrot and celery to the pot. Pour in chicken broth and bring to a boil.
3. Add boneless, skinless chicken breasts to the pot. Reduce heat and simmer for 20-25 minutes, or until chicken is cooked through.
4. Remove chicken breasts from the pot, shred with forks, and return to the pot.
5. Stir in uncooked egg noodles and cook for 8-10 minutes, or until noodles are tender.
6. Season with salt and pepper to taste.

Per serving
Calories: 300| Carbs: 20g| Fats: 8g| Protein: 30g

Beef and Vegetable Soup

Time: 50 minutes| Difficulty: Moderate| Serving 2

4 cups beef broth
8 ounces beef stew meat, cubed
2 carrots, sliced
2 celery stalks, sliced
1 onion, chopped
2 garlic cloves, minced
1/4 cup chopped fresh parsley **and** *2 tablespoons olive oil*

1. Heat olive oil in a large pot over medium heat. Add chopped onion and minced garlic, cook until softened.
2. Add cubed beef stew meat to the pot. Cook until browned on all sides.
3. Pour in beef broth and bring to a boil. Reduce heat and simmer for 30-35 minutes, or until beef is tender.
4. Add sliced carrots and celery to the pot. Cook for an additional 10-15 minutes, or until vegetables are tender.
5. Season with salt and pepper to taste.
6. Stir in chopped fresh parsley.

Per Serving
Calories: 300| Carbs: 15g| Fats: 15g| Protein: 25g

Italian Wedding Soup

Time: 50 minutes| Difficulty: Moderate| Serving 2

4 cups chicken broth
8 ounces ground turkey
1/4 cup uncooked orzo pasta
1 carrot, sliced
1 celery stalk, sliced
1/2 onion, chopped
2 garlic cloves, minced
1/4 cup chopped fresh parsley
1 tablespoon olive oil
Salt and pepper to taste

1. Heat olive oil in a large pot over medium heat. Add chopped onion and minced garlic, cook until softened.
2. Add ground turkey to the pot. Cook until browned, breaking it apart with a spoon.
3. Pour in chicken broth and bring to a boil. Add sliced carrot and celery to the pot.
4. Stir in uncooked orzo pasta. Reduce heat and simmer for 10-12 minutes, or until pasta is cooked through.
5. Stir in chopped fresh parsley.

Per serving
Calories: 250| Carbs: 20g| Fats: 10g| Protein: 20g

Egg Drop Soup

Time: 20 minutes| Difficulty: Easy | Serving 2

4 cups chicken broth

2 eggs, beaten

2 green onions, thinly sliced

1 teaspoon grated ginger

1 tablespoon soy sauce

Salt and pepper to taste

1. Bring chicken broth to a simmer in a large pot.
2. Stir in grated ginger and soy sauce.
3. Slowly pour beaten eggs into the simmering broth while stirring gently with a fork. Cook for 1-2 minutes until eggs are cooked through.
4. Stir in sliced green onions.
5. Season with salt and pepper to taste

Per serving : Calories: 100| Carbs: 5g| Fats: 6g| Protein: 8g

Savory Beef Stew

Time: 1 hour| Difficulty: Medium| Serving 2

1 lb. beef stew meat, cubed

1 onion, chopped

3 cups beef broth

2 carrots, chopped

2 potatoes, diced

1 cup green peas

2 cloves garlic, minced

2 tbsp. olive oil

Salt and pepper to taste

1. Sauté onion and garlic until softened. Add beef and cook until browned.
2. Pour in beef broth and bring to a boil. Reduce heat and simmer for 30 minutes.
3. Add carrots, potatoes, and green peas. Simmer for another 20 minutes until vegetables are tender.
4. Season with salt and pepper before serving.

Per serving: Calories: 280| Protein: 22g| Fat: 10g| Carbs: 25g

Holiday Spinach and Potato Soup

Time: 45 minutes| Difficulty: Easy| Serving 2

2 potatoes, peeled and diced

2 cups spinach, chopped

1 onion, diced

3 cups vegetable broth

1/2 cup coconut milk

2 cloves garlic, minced

2 tbsp. olive oil

Salt and pepper to taste

1. Sauté onion and garlic until softened.
2. Add potatoes and vegetable broth. Simmer until potatoes are cooked.
3. Stir in spinach and coconut milk. Cook until spinach wilts.
4. Blend half of the soup until smooth, then return to the pot.
5. Season with salt and pepper.

Per serving: Calories: 150| Protein: 3g| Fat: 6g| Carbs: 22g

2.4 Meat-based Recipes

Turkey and Avocado Wrap with Whole Wheat Tortilla

Time: 10 minutes| Difficulty: Easy| Serving 2

2 whole wheat tortillas
6 slices of turkey breast
1 avocado, sliced
1/2 cup shredded lettuce
1/4 cup sliced cucumber
2 tablespoons Greek yogurt
1 tablespoon Dijon mustard / Salt and pepper to taste

1. Lay out the whole wheat tortillas on a clean surface.
2. Spread Greek yogurt and Dijon mustard evenly over each tortilla.
3. Place three slices of turkey breast on each tortilla.
4. Arrange avocado slices, shredded lettuce, and sliced cucumber over the turkey.
5. Season with salt and pepper to taste.
6. Roll up the tortillas tightly, folding in the sides as you go.
7. Slice each wrap in half diagonally.
8. Serve immediately or wrap in parchment paper for later.

Per serving: Calories: 300| Carbs: 25g| Fats: 15g| Protein: 20g

Chicken and Vegetable Kabobs with Quinoa

Time: 40 minutes| Difficulty: Moderate| Serving 2

2 boneless, skinless chicken breasts cut into cubes
1 zucchini, sliced
1 bell pepper, cut into chunks
1 red onion, cut into chunks
8 cherry tomatoes
1 cup quinoa
2 cups vegetable broth
2 tablespoons olive oil
2 tablespoons balsamic vinegar
2 cloves garlic, minced
1 teaspoon dried oregano / Salt and pepper to taste
Wooden skewers, soaked in water for 30 minutes

1. In a small bowl, whisk together olive oil, balsamic vinegar, minced garlic, dried oregano, salt, and pepper to make the marinade.
2. Place the chicken cubes in a shallow dish and pour half of the marinade over them. Toss to coat evenly, then cover and refrigerate for at least 15 minutes.
3. In the meantime, cook quinoa according to package instructions, using vegetable broth instead of water for added flavor.
4. Preheat grill or grill pan to medium-high heat.
5. Thread marinated chicken cubes, sliced zucchini, bell pepper chunks, red onion chunks, and cherry tomatoes onto the soaked wooden skewers, alternating between the ingredients.
6. Brush the assembled skewers with the remaining marinade.
7. Grill the kabobs for 8-10 minutes, turning occasionally, until the chicken is cooked through and the vegetables are charred and tender.
8. Serve the chicken and vegetable kabobs hot over a bed of cooked quinoa.

Per serving: Calories: 400| Carbs: 40g| Fats: 10g| Protein: 35g

Turkey and Vegetable Skewers with Quinoa

Time: 30 minutes| Difficulty: Moderate| Serving 2

2 turkey breasts, cut into cubes
1 zucchini, sliced
1 bell pepper, cut into chunks
1 onion, cut into chunks
8 cherry tomatoes
1 cup quinoa
2 cups vegetable broth
2 tablespoons olive oil
2 tablespoons balsamic vinegar
2 cloves garlic, minced
1 teaspoon dried oregano
Salt and pepper to taste
Wooden skewers, soaked in water for 30 minutes

1. In a small bowl, whisk together olive oil, balsamic vinegar, minced garlic, dried oregano, salt, and pepper to make the marinade.
2. Place the turkey cubes in a shallow dish and pour half of the marinade over them. Toss to coat evenly, then cover and refrigerate for at least 15 minutes.
3. In the meantime, cook quinoa according to package instructions, using vegetable broth instead of water for added flavor.
4. Preheat grill or grill pan to medium-high heat.
5. Thread marinated turkey cubes, sliced zucchini, bell pepper chunks, onion chunks, and cherry tomatoes onto the soaked wooden skewers, alternating between the ingredients.
6. Brush the assembled skewers with the remaining marinade.
7. Grill the skewers for 8-10 minutes, turning occasionally, until the turkey is cooked through and the vegetables are charred and tender.
8. Serve the turkey and vegetable skewers hot over a bed of cooked quinoa.

Per 1/2 of the recipe
Calories: 400| Carbs: 40g| Fats: 10g| Protein: 35

Pork Tenderloin with Apple Compote

Time: 40 minutes| Difficulty: Moderate| Serving 2

1 pork tenderloin (about 1 pound)
2 tablespoons olive oil
2 apples, peeled, cored, and diced
*1/4 cup apple cider vinegar **and** 2 tablespoons honey*
1/2 teaspoon ground cinnamon

1. Preheat oven to 375°F (190°C).
2. Season pork tenderloin with salt and pepper.
3. Heat olive oil in an oven-safe skillet over medium-high heat.
4. Sear pork tenderloin on all sides until browned, about 2-3 minutes per side.
5. Transfer skillet to the preheated oven and roast pork tenderloin for 20-25 minutes, or until cooked through and internal temperature reaches 145°F (63°C).

In the meantime, prepare the apple compote: In a saucepan, combine diced apples, apple cider vinegar, honey, and ground cinnamon. Cook over medium heat until apples are soft and mixture has thickened.

Serve sliced pork tenderloin with apple compote on the side.

Per Serving
Calories: 300| Carbs: 20g| Fats: 10g| Protein: 25g

Chicken Fajitas

Time: 30 minutes| Difficulty: Easy| Serving 2

2 boneless, skinless chicken breasts, sliced
1 bell pepper, sliced
1 onion, sliced
1 tablespoon olive oil
2 tablespoons fajita seasoning
8 small whole wheat tortillas

Optional toppings: *shredded lettuce, diced tomatoes, shredded cheese, Greek yogurt*

1. Heat olive oil in a skillet over medium-high heat.
2. Add sliced chicken breasts to the skillet and sprinkle with fajita seasoning. Cook until chicken is browned and cooked through, about 5-7 minutes.
3. Add sliced bell pepper and onion to the skillet and cook until vegetables are tender, about 3-4 minutes.
4. Warm whole wheat tortillas in the microwave or on a skillet.
5. Serve chicken and vegetable mixture in warmed tortillas, topped with optional toppings as desired.

Per serving 2 fajitas with toppings
Calories: 350| Carbs: 30g| Fats: 10g|Protein: 30g

Turkey and Cranberry Wrap

Time: 10 minutes| Difficulty: Easy| Serving 2

2 whole wheat tortillas
6 slices of turkey breast
2 tablespoons cranberry sauce
1/4 cup shredded lettuce
1/4 cup sliced cucumber
2 tablespoons Greek yogurt (optional)

1. Lay out the whole wheat tortillas on a clean surface.
2. Spread a tablespoon of cranberry sauce evenly over each tortilla.
3. Place three slices of turkey breast on each tortilla.
4. Arrange shredded lettuce and sliced cucumber over the turkey.
5. If desired, spread a tablespoon of Greek yogurt over the ingredients.
6. Season with salt and pepper to taste.
7. Roll up the tortillas tightly, folding in the sides as you go.
8. Slice each wrap in half diagonally.
9. Serve immediately or wrap in parchment paper for later

Per serving 1 wrap
Calories: 250| Carbs: 25g| Fats: 5g|Protein: 20g

Turkey and Spinach Stuffed Bell Peppers

Time: 45 minutes| Difficulty: Moderate| Serving 2

4 bell peppers, halved and seeded
1 pound ground turkey
1 cup cooked quinoa
1 cup spinach, chopped
1/2 cup shredded mozzarella cheese
1/4 cup chopped fresh parsley
1 teaspoon dried Italian seasoning
1 cup tomato sauce

1. Preheat oven to 375°F (190°C). Arrange bell pepper halves in a baking dish.
2. In a skillet, cook ground turkey until browned. Drain excess fat.
3. In a large bowl, combine cooked ground turkey, cooked quinoa, chopped spinach, shredded mozzarella cheese, chopped parsley, dried Italian seasoning, salt, and pepper. Mix well.
4. Spoon the turkey and spinach mixture into the bell pepper halves.
5. Pour tomato sauce over the stuffed bell peppers.
6. Cover the baking dish with foil and bake in the preheated oven for 30-35 minutes, or until peppers are tenders.
7. Serve hot, garnished with additional parsley if desired.

Per 1 stuffed bell pepper half
Calories: 250| Carbs: 15g| Fats: 10g| Protein: 25g

Baked Lemon Herb Chicken

Time: 30 minutes| Difficulty: Easy| Serving 2

2 boneless, skinless chicken breasts
1 lemon, thinly sliced
2 cloves garlic, minced
1 tablespoon fresh rosemary, chopped
1 tablespoon fresh thyme, chopped
Salt and pepper to taste
1 tablespoon olive oil

1. Preheat your oven to 375°F (190°C).
2. In a small bowl, mix together the minced garlic, chopped rosemary, chopped thyme, salt, pepper, and olive oil.
3. Place the chicken breasts in a baking dish. Rub the herb mixture over both sides of the chicken breasts.
4. Arrange the lemon slices on top of the chicken breasts.
5. Cover the baking dish with foil and bake in the preheated oven for 25-30 minutes, or until the chicken is cooked through and no longer pink in the center.
6. Remove the foil during the last 5 minutes of baking to allow the chicken to brown slightly.
7. Serve the baked lemon herb chicken hot, garnished with additional fresh herbs if desired.

Per serving
Calories: 250| Protein: 30g| Carbs: 4g| Fat: 12g| Fiber: 1g

Beef Stir-Fry with Vegetables

Time: 30 minutes| Difficulty: Easy| Serving 2

8 ounces beef sirloin, thinly sliced
1 tablespoon soy sauce
1 tablespoon oyster sauce
1 tablespoon olive oil
2 cloves garlic, minced
1 bell pepper, sliced
1 onion, sliced
1 cup broccoli florets
Cooked rice or quinoa for serving

1. In a bowl, marinate beef slices with soy sauce and oyster sauce for 10-15 minutes.
2. Heat olive oil in a skillet or wok over medium-high heat.
3. Add minced garlic and stir-fry for 30 seconds.
4. Add marinated beef slices and stir-fry until browned, about 2-3 minutes.
5. Add sliced bell pepper, onion, and broccoli florets to the skillet. Stir-fry for an additional 3-4 minutes, or until vegetables are tender-crisp.
6. Serve hot over cooked rice or quinoa.

Per 1/2 of the recipe without rice/quinoa
Calories: 300| Carbs: 10g| Fats: 15g| Protein: 25g

Pork Tenderloin with Honey Mustard Glaze

Time: 35 minutes| Difficulty: Easy| Serving 2

1 pork tenderloin (about 1 pound)
2 tablespoons Dijon mustard
1 tablespoon honey
1 tablespoon olive oil
2 cloves garlic, minced
Salt and pepper to taste

1. Preheat oven to 375°F (190°C).
2. In a small bowl, whisk together Dijon mustard, honey, olive oil, minced garlic, salt, and pepper to make the glaze.
3. Place pork tenderloin on a baking sheet lined with parchment paper.
4. Brush the glaze over the pork tenderloin, coating it evenly.
5. Bake in the preheated oven for 25-30 minutes, or until pork is cooked through and internal temperature reaches 145°F (63°C).
6. Let the pork rest for 5 minutes before slicing.
7. Serve hot with roasted vegetables or a side salad.

Per 4 oz. pork tenderloin
Calories: 200| Carbs: 5g| Fats: 10g| Protein: 25g

Lamb Chops with Mint Yogurt Sauce

Time: 35 minutes| Difficulty: Moderate| Serving 2

4 lamb chops
2 tablespoons olive oil
2 cloves garlic, minced
1 tablespoon chopped fresh rosemary
Salt and pepper to taste
1/2 cup Greek yogurt
1 tablespoon chopped fresh mint
1 tablespoon lemon juice

1. Preheat grill to medium-high heat.
2. Rub lamb chops with olive oil, minced garlic, chopped rosemary, salt, and pepper.
3. Grill lamb chops for 4-5 minutes on each side, or until cooked to desired doneness.
4. In a small bowl, mix together Greek yogurt, chopped mint, and lemon juice to make the mint yogurt sauce.
5. Serve hot lamb chops with mint yogurt sauce on the side.

Per 1 lamb chop with sauce
Calories: 300| Carbs: 2g| Fats: 20g| Protein: 25g

Turkey Meatballs in Tomato Sauce

Time: 40 minutes| Difficulty: Easy| Serving 2

1 pound ground turkey
1/4 cup breadcrumbs
1 egg
2 cloves garlic, minced
1/4 cup grated Parmesan cheese
1 tablespoon chopped fresh parsley
Salt and pepper to taste
2 cups tomato sauce

1. Preheat oven to 375°F (190°C). Line a baking sheet with parchment paper.
2. In a bowl, combine ground turkey, breadcrumbs, egg, minced garlic, Parmesan cheese, chopped parsley, salt, and pepper. Mix until well combined.
3. Shape the mixture into small meatballs and place them on the prepared baking sheet.
4. Bake in the preheated oven for 20-25 minutes, or until meatballs are cooked through and golden brown.
5. Meanwhile, heat tomato sauce in a saucepan over medium heat.
6. Once meatballs are cooked, add them to the tomato sauce and simmer for 5-10 minutes.
7. Serve hot with your choice of side dishes.

Per 4 meatballs with sauce
Calories: 300| Carbs: 10g| Fats: 15g| Protein: 25g

Beef and Mushroom Skewers

Time: 30 minutes| Difficulty: Moderate| Serving 2

1 pound beef sirloin, cut into cubes
1 cup mushrooms, sliced
1 red bell pepper, cut into chunks
1 onion, cut into chunks
2 tablespoons olive oil
2 cloves garlic, minced
1 tablespoon Worcestershire sauce
Salt and pepper to taste

1. In a bowl, combine beef cubes, sliced mushrooms, red bell pepper chunks, onion chunks, olive oil, minced garlic, Worcestershire sauce, salt, and pepper. Mix well to coat.
2. Thread the beef, mushrooms, bell pepper, and onion onto skewers.
3. Preheat grill to medium-high heat.
4. Grill skewers for 8-10 minutes, turning occasionally, until beef is cooked to desired doneness and vegetables are tender.
5. Serve hot with your favorite side dish.

Per 1/4 of the recipe
Calories: 300| Carbs: 5g| Fats: 15g| Protein: 30g

Lamb Kebabs with Yogurt Sauce

Time: 30 minutes| Difficulty: Moderate| Serving 2

1 pound lamb cubes
1/4 cup olive oil
2 cloves garlic, minced
1 tablespoon lemon juice
1 teaspoon ground cumin
1 teaspoon paprika
Wooden skewers, soaked in water for 30 minutes
1/2 cup Greek yogurt
1 tablespoon chopped fresh mint
1 tablespoon chopped fresh parsley

1. In a bowl, mix together olive oil, minced garlic, lemon juice, ground cumin, paprika, salt, and pepper to make the marinade.
2. Thread lamb cubes onto the soaked wooden skewers.
3. Brush the marinade over the lamb kebabs.
4. Grill kebabs for 8-10 minutes, turning occasionally, until lamb is cooked through.
5. In a small bowl, mix together Greek yogurt, chopped mint, and chopped parsley to make the yogurt sauce.
6. Serve hot lamb kebabs with yogurt sauce on the side.

Per 1/2 of the recipe without sauce
Calories: 350| Carbs: 2g| Fats: 25g\ Protein: 30g

Turkey Chili

Time: 45 minutes| Difficulty: Easy| Serving 2

1 tbs. olive oil
1 onion, chopped
2 cloves garlic, minced
1 pound ground turkey
1 bell pepper, diced
1 can (14 ounces) diced tomatoes
1 can (14 ounces) kidney beans, drained and rinsed
1 cup vegetable broth
*2 tablespoons chili powder **and** 1 teaspoon ground cumin*
***Optional toppings:** shredded cheese, diced avocado, Greek yogurt*

1. Heat olive oil in a large pot over medium heat.
2. Add chopped onion and minced garlic, and sauté until softened.
3. Add ground turkey to the pot and cook until browned.
4. Stir in diced bell pepper, diced tomatoes, kidney beans, vegetable broth, chili powder, ground cumin, salt, and pepper.
5. Bring chili to a simmer and let cook for 30 minutes, stirring occasionally.
6. Serve hot, topped with shredded cheese, diced avocado, and Greek yogurt if desired.

Per Serving
Calories: 250| Carbs: 15g| Fats: 10g| Protein: 20g

Grilled Steak with Chimichurri Sauce

Time: 40 minutes| Difficulty: Moderate| Serving 2

2 beef
2 tablespoons olive oil
2 cloves garlic, minced
1/4 cup chopped fresh parsley
2 tablespoons chopped fresh cilantro
2 tablespoons red wine vinegar
1/2 teaspoon dried oregano

1. Preheat grill to medium-high heat.
2. Season steaks with salt and pepper.
3. In a small bowl, mix together olive oil, minced garlic, chopped parsley, chopped cilantro, red wine vinegar, dried oregano, salt, and pepper to make the chimichurri.
4. Grill steaks for 4-6 minutes on each side, or until desired doneness.
5. Let steaks rest for 5 minutes before slicing.
6. Serve hot with chimichurri sauce drizzled over the top.

Per 1 steak with sauce
Calories: 400| Carbs: 2g| Fats: 25g| Protein: 40g

Beef and Bean Chili

Time: 1 hour| Difficulty: Moderate| Serving 2

1 tablespoon olive oil
1 onion, chopped
2 cloves garlic, minced
1 pound ground beef
1 can (14 ounces) diced tomatoes
1 can (14 ounces) kidney beans, drained and rinsed
1 cup beef broth
2 tablespoons chili powder and 1 teaspoon ground cumin
***Optional toppings:** shredded cheese, diced avocado, Greek yogurt*

1. Heat olive oil in a large pot over medium heat.
2. Add chopped onion and minced garlic, and sauté until softened.
3. Add ground beef to the pot and cook until browned.
4. Stir in diced tomatoes, kidney beans, beef broth, chili powder, ground cumin, salt, and pepper.
5. Bring chili to a simmer and let cook for 30-40 minutes, stirring occasionally.
6. Serve hot, topped with optional toppings as desired.

Per 1/6 of the recipe without toppings
Calories: 300| Carbs: 15g| Fats: 15g| Protein: 25g

Chicken and Broccoli Casserole

Time: 50 minutes| Difficulty: Moderate| Serving 2

2 boneless, skinless chicken breasts, cooked and shredded
2 cups broccoli florets, steamed
1 cup cooked quinoa
1 cup shredded cheddar cheese
1/2 cup Greek yogurt
1/4 cup milk
2 cloves garlic, minced
Salt and pepper to taste
1/4 cup breadcrumbs (optional)

1. Preheat oven to 375°F (190°C). Grease a casserole dish.
2. In a large bowl, combine cooked and shredded chicken, steamed broccoli florets, cooked quinoa, shredded cheddar cheese, Greek yogurt, milk, minced garlic, salt, and pepper. Mix well.
3. Transfer the mixture to the prepared casserole dish and spread evenly.
4. If desired, sprinkle breadcrumbs over the top of the casserole.
5. Bake in the preheated oven for 25-30 minutes, or until bubbly and golden brown on top.
6. Serve hot, garnished with chopped parsley if desired.

Per serving
Calories: 300| Carbs: 20g| Fats: 15g| Protein: 25g

Balsamic Glazed Pork Tenderloin

Time: 40 minutes| Difficulty: Moderate| Serving 2

1 pork tenderloin (about 1 pound)
2 tablespoons olive oil
2 cloves garlic, minced
1/4 cup balsamic vinegar
2 tablespoons honey
1 teaspoon dried thyme

1. Preheat oven to 375°F (190°C).
2. Season pork tenderloin with salt and pepper.
3. In an oven-safe skillet, heat olive oil over medium-high heat.
4. Sear pork tenderloin on all sides until browned, about 2-3 minutes per side.
5. Add minced garlic to the skillet and cook for 1 minute.
6. In a small bowl, whisk together balsamic vinegar, honey, dried thyme, salt, and pepper.
7. Pour the balsamic glaze over the pork tenderloin in the skillet.
8. Transfer the skillet to the preheated oven and roast for 20-25 minutes, or until pork is cooked through.
9. Let the pork rest for 5 minutes before slicing.
10. Serve hot, garnished with fresh parsley.

Per 4 oz. pork tenderloin
Calories: 250| Carbs: 10g| Fats: 10g|Protein: 25g

Pork and Vegetable Stir-Fry

Time: 30 minutes| Difficulty: Easy| Serving 2

1 pound pork loin, thinly sliced
2 tablespoons soy sauce
1 tablespoon oyster sauce
1 tablespoon olive oil
2 cloves garlic, minced
1 bell pepper, sliced
1 cup broccoli florets
1 carrot, julienned

1. In a bowl, marinate pork slices with soy sauce and oyster sauce for 10-15 minutes.
2. Heat olive oil in a skillet or wok over medium-high heat.
3. Add minced garlic and stir-fry for 30 seconds.
4. Add marinated pork slices to the skillet and stir-fry until browned, about 2-3 minutes.
5. Add sliced bell pepper, broccoli florets, and julienned carrot to the skillet. Stir-fry for an additional 3-4 minutes, or until vegetables are tender-crisp.

Per 1/2 of the recipe without rice/quinoa
Calories: 300| Carbs: 10g| Fats: 15g| Protein: 25g

2.5 Fish-based Recipes

Lemon Herb Baked Salmon

Time: 25 minutes| Difficulty: Easy| Serving 2

2 salmon fillets (6 ounces each)
2 tablespoons olive oil
1 tablespoon lemon juice
1 teaspoon lemon zest
2 cloves garlic, minced
1 teaspoon dried thyme
Salt and pepper to taste
Fresh parsley for garnish

1. Preheat oven to 375°F (190°C).
2. In a small bowl, mix together olive oil, lemon juice, lemon zest, minced garlic, dried thyme, salt, and pepper.
3. Place salmon fillets on a baking sheet lined with parchment paper.
4. Brush the salmon fillets with the lemon herb mixture.
5. Bake in the preheated oven for 12-15 minutes, or until the salmon is cooked through and flakes easily with a fork.
6. Garnish with fresh parsley before serving.

Per 1 salmon fillet
Calories: 350| Carbs: 0g| Fats: 20g| Protein: 35g

Lemon Garlic Tilapia

Time: 20 minutes| Difficulty: Easy| Serving 2

2 tilapia fillets (6 ounces each)
2 tablespoons olive oil
2 cloves garlic, minced
1 tablespoon lemon juice
1 teaspoon lemon zest
1 teaspoon dried oregano
Salt and pepper to taste
Fresh parsley for garnish

1. Preheat oven to 375°F (190°C).
2. Place tilapia fillets on a baking sheet lined with parchment paper.
3. In a small bowl, mix together olive oil, minced garlic, lemon juice, lemon zest, dried oregano, salt, and pepper.
4. Brush the tilapia fillets with the lemon garlic mixture.
5. Bake in the preheated oven for 12-15 minutes, or until the tilapia is cooked through and flakes easily with a fork.
6. Garnish with fresh parsley before serving.

Per 1 tilapia fillet: Calories: 250| Carbs: 0g| Fats: 15g| Protein: 30g

Garlic Butter Grilled Shrimp

Time: 20 minutes| Difficulty: Easy| Serving 2

1 pound large shrimp, peeled and deveined
3 tablespoons melted butter
3 cloves garlic, minced
1 tablespoon chopped fresh parsley
1 tablespoon lemon juice
Salt and pepper to taste
Wooden skewers, soaked in water for 30 minutes

1. Preheat grill to medium-high heat.
2. In a bowl, combine melted butter, minced garlic, chopped parsley, lemon juice, salt, and pepper.
3. Thread the shrimp onto the soaked wooden skewers.
4. Brush the shrimp skewers with the garlic butter mixture.
5. Grill the shrimp skewers for 2-3 minutes on each side, or until shrimp are pink and opaque.
6. Serve hot with additional lemon wedges for squeezing.

Per 1/4 of the recipe
Calories: 200| Carbs: 0g| Fats: 10g| Protein: 25g

Pan-Seared Mahi-Mahi with Mango Salsa

Time: 25 minutes| Difficulty: Easy| Serving 2

2 mahi-mahi fillets (6 ounces each)
2 tablespoons olive oil
1 teaspoon paprika
Salt and pepper to taste
1 ripe mango, peeled and diced
1/2 red bell pepper, diced
1/4 red onion, finely chopped
1 tablespoon chopped fresh cilantro
1 tablespoon lime juice

1. Season mahi-mahi fillets with paprika, salt, and pepper.
2. Heat olive oil in a skillet over medium-high heat.
3. Add mahi-mahi fillets to the skillet and cook for 3-4 minutes on each side, or until fish is cooked through and golden brown.
4. In a bowl, combine diced mango, diced red bell pepper, chopped red onion, chopped cilantro, and lime juice to make the salsa.
5. Serve pan-seared mahi-mahi with mango salsa on top.

Per 1 mahi-mahi fillet with salsa
Calories: 300| Carbs: 20g| Fats: 10g| Protein: 30g

Lemon Herb Baked Salmon

Time: 25 minutes| Difficulty: Easy| Serving 2

2 salmon fillets (6 ounces each)
2 tablespoons olive oil
1 tablespoon lemon juice
1 teaspoon lemon zest
2 cloves garlic, minced
1 teaspoon dried thyme
Salt and pepper to taste
Fresh parsley for garnish

7. Preheat oven to 375°F (190°C).
8. In a small bowl, mix together olive oil, lemon juice, lemon zest, minced garlic, dried thyme, salt, and pepper.
9. Place salmon fillets on a baking sheet lined with parchment paper.
10. Brush the salmon fillets with the lemon herb mixture.
11. Bake in the preheated oven for 12-15 minutes, or until the salmon is cooked through and flakes easily with a fork.
12. Garnish with fresh parsley before serving.

Per 1 salmon fillet
Calories: 350| Carbs: 0g| Fats: 20g| Protein: 35g

Lemon Garlic Tilapia

Time: 20 minutes| Difficulty: Easy| Serving 2

2 tilapia fillets (6 ounces each)
2 tablespoons olive oil
2 cloves garlic, minced
1 tablespoon lemon juice
1 teaspoon lemon zest
1 teaspoon dried oregano
Salt and pepper to taste
Fresh parsley for garnish

7. Preheat oven to 375°F (190°C).
8. Place tilapia fillets on a baking sheet lined with parchment paper.
9. In a small bowl, mix together olive oil, minced garlic, lemon juice, lemon zest, dried oregano, salt, and pepper.
10. Brush the tilapia fillets with the lemon garlic mixture.
11. Bake in the preheated oven for 12-15 minutes, or until the tilapia is cooked through and flakes easily with a fork.
12. Garnish with fresh parsley before serving.

Per 1 tilapia fillet
Calories: 250| Carbs: 0g| Fats: 15g| Protein: 30g

Garlic Butter Grilled Shrimp

Time: 20 minutes| Difficulty: Easy| Serving 2

1 pound large shrimp, peeled and deveined
3 tablespoons melted butter
3 cloves garlic, minced
1 tablespoon chopped fresh parsley
1 tablespoon lemon juice
Salt and pepper to taste
Wooden skewers, soaked in water for 30 minutes

7. Preheat grill to medium-high heat.
8. In a bowl, combine melted butter, minced garlic, chopped parsley, lemon juice, salt, and pepper.
9. Thread the shrimp onto the soaked wooden skewers.
10. Brush the shrimp skewers with the garlic butter mixture.
11. Grill the shrimp skewers for 2-3 minutes on each side, or until shrimp are pink and opaque.
12. Serve hot with additional lemon wedges for squeezing.

Per 1/4 of the recipe
Calories: 200| Carbs: 0g| Fats: 10g| Protein: 25g

Pan-Seared Mahi-Mahi with Mango Salsa

Time: 25 minutes| Difficulty: Easy| Serving 2

2 mahi-mahi fillets (6 ounces each)
2 tablespoons olive oil
1 teaspoon paprika
Salt and pepper to taste
1 ripe mango, peeled and diced
1/2 red bell pepper, diced
1/4 red onion, finely chopped
1 tablespoon chopped fresh cilantro
1 tablespoon lime juice

6. Season mahi-mahi fillets with paprika, salt, and pepper.
7. Heat olive oil in a skillet over medium-high heat.
8. Add mahi-mahi fillets to the skillet and cook for 3-4 minutes on each side, or until fish is cooked through and golden brown.
9. In a bowl, combine diced mango, diced red bell pepper, chopped red onion, chopped cilantro, and lime juice to make the salsa.
10. Serve pan-seared mahi-mahi with mango salsa on top.

Per 1 mahi-mahi fillet with salsa
Calories: 300| Carbs: 20g| Fats: 10g| Protein: 30g

Grilled Swordfish with Mango Salsa

Time: 25 minutes| Difficulty: Easy| Serving 2

2 swordfish steaks (6 ounces each)
2 tablespoons olive oil
1 teaspoon paprika
1/2 teaspoon ground cumin
Salt and pepper to taste
1 ripe mango, peeled and diced
1/2 red onion, finely chopped
1 jalapeño, seeded and minced
2 tablespoons chopped fresh cilantro
1 tablespoon lime juice

1.   Preheat grill to medium-high heat.
2.   Brush swordfish steaks with olive oil and season with paprika, ground cumin, salt, and pepper.
3.   Grill swordfish steaks for 4-5 minutes on each side, or until fish is cooked through and has grill marks.
4.   In a bowl, combine diced mango, chopped red onion, minced jalapeño, chopped cilantro, and lime juice to make the salsa.
5.   Serve grilled swordfish steaks with mango salsa on top.

Per 1 swordfish steak with salsa
Calories: 300| Carbs: 15g| Fats: 15g| Protein: 30g

Grilled Halibut with Asparagus

Time: 25 minutes| Difficulty: Easy| Serving 2

2 halibut fillets (6 ounces each)
2 tablespoons olive oil
2 cloves garlic, minced
1 tablespoon lemon juice
1 bunch asparagus, trimmed
Lemon wedges for serving

1.   Preheat grill to medium-high heat.
2.   In a small bowl, mix together olive oil, minced garlic, lemon juice, salt, and pepper.
3.   Brush halibut fillets with the olive oil mixture.
4.   Place halibut fillets and asparagus on the grill.
5.   Grill halibut for 4-5 minutes on each side, or until fish is cooked through and flakes easily with a fork.
6.   Grill asparagus for 3-4 minutes, or until tender-crisp.
7.   Serve grilled halibut and asparagus hot with lemon wedges on the side.

Per 1 halibut fillet with asparagus
Calories: 300| Carbs: 5g| Fats: 15g| Protein: 35

Baked Cod with Tomato and Olive Relish

Time: 30 minutes| Difficulty: Easy| Serving 2

2 cod fillets (6 ounces each)
1 tablespoon olive oil
2 cloves garlic, minced
1 cup cherry tomatoes, halved
1/4 cup pitted olives, chopped
1 tablespoon capers
1 tablespoon chopped fresh parsley
Salt and pepper to taste
Lemon wedges for serving

1. Preheat oven to 375°F (190°C).
2. Place cod fillets on a baking sheet lined with parchment paper.
3. In a small bowl, mix together olive oil, minced garlic, cherry tomatoes, chopped olives, capers, chopped parsley, salt, and pepper.
4. Spoon the tomato and olive relish over the cod fillets.
5. Bake in the preheated oven for 15-18 minutes, or until the cod is cooked through and flakes easily with a fork.
6. Serve hot with lemon wedges on the side.

Per 1 cod fillet with relish
Calories: 250| Carbs: 5g| Fats: 10g| Protein: 35g

Mediterranean Baked Cod

Time: 25 minutes| Difficulty: Easy| Serving 2

2 cod fillets (6 ounces each)
2 tablespoons olive oil
2 cloves garlic, minced
1 teaspoon dried oregano
1 teaspoon dried thyme
1/2 cup cherry tomatoes, halved
1/4 cup pitted olives, chopped
1/4 cup crumbled feta cheese

1. Preheat oven to 375°F (190°C).
2. Place cod fillets on a baking sheet lined with parchment paper.
3. In a small bowl, mix together olive oil, minced garlic, dried oregano, dried thyme, salt, and pepper.
4. Brush the cod fillets with the olive oil mixture.
5. Arrange cherry tomatoes and chopped olives around the cod fillets on the baking sheet.
6. Bake in the preheated oven for 15-18 minutes, or until the cod is cooked through and flakes easily with a fork.
7. Sprinkle crumbled feta cheese over the baked cod and garnish with fresh parsley before serving.

Per 1 cod fillet
Calories: 300| Carbs: 5g| Fats: 15g| Protein: 30g

Lemon Garlic Baked Cod

Time: 20 minutes| Difficulty: Easy| Serving 2

2 cod fillets (6 ounces each)
2 tablespoons olive oil
2 cloves garlic, minced
1 tablespoon lemon juice
1 teaspoon lemon zest
Chopped fresh parsley for garnish

1. Preheat oven to 375°F (190°C).
2. Place cod fillets on a baking sheet lined with parchment paper.
3. In a small bowl, mix together olive oil, minced garlic, lemon juice, lemon zest, salt, and pepper.
4. Brush the cod fillets with the lemon garlic mixture.
5. Bake in the preheated oven for 12-15 minutes, or until the cod is cooked through and flakes easily with a fork.
6. Garnish with chopped fresh parsley before serving.

Per 1 cod fillet
Calories: 200| Carbs: 0g| Fats: 10g| Protein: 30g

Coconut Curry Shrimp

Time: 30 minutes| Difficulty: Moderate| Serving 2

1 pound large shrimp, peeled and deveined
1 tablespoon olive oil
2 cloves garlic, minced
1 tablespoon curry powder
1 can (14 ounces) coconut milk
1 red bell pepper, sliced
1 cup snap peas
Salt and pepper to taste
Cooked rice for serving
Chopped fresh cilantro for garnish

1. Heat olive oil in a skillet over medium heat.
2. Add minced garlic and curry powder to the skillet, and cook for 1 minute.
3. Stir in coconut milk, sliced red bell pepper, and snap peas. Simmer for 5 minutes.
4. Add shrimp to the skillet and cook for 3-4 minutes, or until shrimp are pink and cooked through.
5. Season with salt and pepper to taste.
6. Serve coconut curry shrimp over cooked rice, garnished with chopped fresh cilantro.

Per 1/4 of the recipe without rice)
Calories: 250| Carbs: 10g| Fats: 15g| Protein: 25g

Teriyaki Glazed Salmon

Time: 30 minutes| Difficulty: Easy| Serving 2

2 salmon fillets (6 ounces each)
1/4 cup soy sauce (or tamari for gluten-free)
2 tablespoons honey
1 tablespoon rice vinegar
1 clove garlic, minced
1 teaspoon minced ginger
1 teaspoon sesame oil
Sesame seeds and sliced green onions for garnish

1. In a small saucepan, combine soy sauce, honey, rice vinegar, minced garlic, minced ginger, and sesame oil. Heat over medium heat and simmer until the sauce thickens slightly, about 5-7 minutes.
2. Preheat the grill or grill pan to medium-high heat.
3. Brush the salmon fillets with the teriyaki sauce and grill for 4-5 minutes on each side, or until the salmon is cooked through and flakes easily with a fork.
4. Serve hot, garnished with sesame seeds and sliced green onions.

Per 1 salmon fillet
Calories: 350| Carbs: 15g| Fats: 20g Protein: 30g

Coconut Lime Shrimp Skewers

Time: 20 minutes| Difficulty: Easy| Serving 2

1 pound large shrimp, peeled and deveined
1/4 cup coconut milk
Zest and juice of 1 lime
2 tablespoons chopped fresh cilantro
1 tablespoon olive oil
Salt and pepper to taste
Wooden skewers, soaked in water for 30 minutes

1. In a bowl, combine coconut milk, lime zest, lime juice, chopped cilantro, olive oil, salt, and pepper to make the marinade.
2. Thread shrimp onto the soaked wooden skewers.
3. Brush shrimp skewers with the coconut lime marinade.
4. Preheat the grill or grill pan to medium-high heat.
5. Grill shrimp skewers for 2-3 minutes on each side, or until shrimp are pink and cooked through.

Per 1/4 of the recipe
Calories: 150| Carbs: 1g| Fats: 5g| Protein: 25g

Pan-Seared Sea Bass with Citrus Salsa

Time: 25 minutes| Difficulty: Easy| Serving 2

2 sea bass fillets (6 ounces each)
2 tablespoons olive oil
Salt and pepper to taste
1 orange, segmented
1 grapefruit, segmented
1/4 red onion, finely chopped
1 tablespoon chopped fresh cilantro
1 tablespoon lime juice
1 tablespoon honey

1. Heat olive oil in a skillet over medium-high heat.
2. Season sea bass fillets with salt and pepper.
3. Sear sea bass fillets for 3-4 minutes on each side, or until fish is golden brown and cooked through.
4. In a bowl, combine orange segments, grapefruit segments, chopped red onion, chopped cilantro, lime juice, and honey to make the salsa.
5. Serve pan-seared sea bass with citrus salsa on top.

Per 1 sea bass fillet with salsa
Calories: 300| Carbs: 20g| Fats: 10g| Protein: 30g

Cajun Spiced Catfish

Time: 25 minutes| Difficulty: Easy| Serving 2

2 catfish fillets (6 ounces each)
2 tablespoons olive oil
1 tablespoon Cajun seasoning
1 teaspoon paprika
1/2 teaspoon garlic powder
1/2 teaspoon onion powder
Salt and pepper to taste
Lemon wedges for serving

1. Preheat oven to 375°F (190°C).
2. Rub catfish fillets with olive oil and season with Cajun seasoning, paprika, garlic powder, onion powder, salt, and pepper.
3. Heat olive oil in a skillet over medium-high heat.
4. Sear catfish fillets for 2-3 minutes on each side until browned.
5. Transfer catfish fillets to a baking dish and bake in the preheated oven for 10-12 minutes, or until fish are cooked through and flakes easily with a fork.
6. Serve hot with lemon wedges on the side.

Per 1 catfish fillet
Calories: 300| Carbs: 5g| Fats: 15g| Protein: 35g

Honey Garlic Glazed Salmon

Time: 30 minutes| Difficulty: Easy| Serving 2
2 salmon fillets (6 ounces each)
2 tablespoons honey
2 tablespoons soy sauce
1 tablespoon olive oil
2 cloves garlic, minced
1 teaspoon grated ginger / Sesame seeds for garnish
Sliced green onions for garnish
1. In a small bowl, whisk together honey, soy sauce, minced garlic, and grated ginger to make the glaze.
2. Heat olive oil in a skillet over medium-high heat.
3. Season salmon fillets with salt and pepper, then place them skin-side down in the skillet.
4. Cook salmon for 3-4 minutes on each side, or until browned and cooked through.
5. Brush salmon fillets with the honey garlic glaze during the last minute of cooking.
6. Sprinkle sesame seeds and sliced green onions over the glazed salmon before serving.

Per 1 salmon fillet
Calories: 350| Carbs: 15g| Fats: 20g| Protein: 30g

Baked Salmon with Garlic and Herbs

Time: 25 minutes| Difficulty: Easy| Serving 2
2 salmon fillets
2 tablespoons olive oil
2 cloves garlic, minced
1 tablespoon chopped fresh parsley
1 teaspoon dried thyme
1. Preheat oven to 375°F (190°C).
2. Place salmon fillets on a baking sheet lined with parchment paper.
3. In a small bowl, mix together olive oil, minced garlic, chopped parsley, dried thyme, salt, and pepper.
4. Spread the garlic and herb mixture evenly over the salmon fillets.
5. Bake in the preheated oven for 12-15 minutes, or until salmon is cooked through and flakes easily with a fork.
6. Serve hot with steamed vegetables or a side salad.

Per 1 salmon fillet
Calories: 250| Carbs: 0g| Fats: 15g| Protein: 25g

Lemon Pepper Tuna Steaks

Time: 20 minutes| Difficulty: Easy| Serving 2
2 tuna steaks (6 ounces each)
2 tablespoons olive oil
Zest and juice of 1 lemon
1 teaspoon cracked black pepper / Salt to taste
Fresh parsley for garnish
1. Preheat grill or grill pan to medium-high heat.
2. In a small bowl, mix together olive oil, lemon zest, lemon juice, cracked black pepper, and salt.
3. Brush both sides of the tuna steaks with the lemon pepper mixture.
4. Grill tuna steaks for 3-4 minutes on each side, or until desired doneness.
5. Serve hot, garnished with fresh parsley.

Per 1 tuna steak
Calories: 250| Carbs: 0g| Fats: 15g| Protein: 30g

Pesto Baked Cod

Time: 20 minutes| Difficulty: Easy| Serving 2

2 cod fillets (6 ounces each)
2 tablespoons prepared pesto
1 tablespoon olive oil
Fresh basil leaves for garnish

1. Preheat oven to 375°F (190°C).
2. Place cod fillets on a baking sheet lined with parchment paper.
3. Spread a tablespoon of prepared pesto over each cod fillet.
4. Drizzle olive oil over the pesto-coated cod fillets.
5. Season cod fillets with salt and pepper to taste.
6. Bake in the preheated oven for 12-15 minutes, or until the cod is cooked through and flakes easily with a fork.
7. Garnish with fresh basil leaves before serving.

Per 1 cod fillet
Calories: 250| Carbs: 2g| Fats: 15g| Protein: 30g

Asian-Inspired Salmon Salad

Time: 30 minutes| Difficulty: Easy| Serving 2

2 salmon fillets (6 ounces each)
2 tablespoons soy sauce
1 tablespoon sesame oil
1 tablespoon rice vinegar
1 teaspoon grated ginger
1 teaspoon honey
Mixed salad greens
Sliced cucumber
Sliced bell peppers
Sliced radishes

1. Preheat oven to 375°F (190°C).
2. In a small bowl, whisk together soy sauce, sesame oil, rice vinegar, grated ginger, and honey.
3. Place salmon fillets on a baking sheet lined with parchment paper.
4. Brush salmon fillets with the soy sauce mixture.
5. Bake in the preheated oven for 12-15 minutes, or until salmon is cooked through and flakes easily with a fork.
6. Arrange mixed salad greens, sliced cucumber, sliced bell peppers, and sliced radishes on plates.
7. Place baked salmon fillets on top of the salad.

Per 1 salmon fillet with salad
Calories: 350| Carbs: 15g| Fats: 20g| Protein: 30g

2.6 Side Dishes

Quinoa Pilaf

Time: 30 minutes| Difficulty: Easy| Serving 2

1 cup quinoa
2 cups vegetable broth
1 tablespoon olive oil
1 onion, diced
2 cloves garlic, minced
1 carrot, diced
1 bell pepper, diced
1/2 cup frozen peas
Salt and pepper to taste
Fresh parsley for garnish

1. Rinse quinoa under cold water, and then combine with vegetable broth in a saucepan. Bring to a boil, then reduce heat to low, cover, and simmer for 15-20 minutes, or until quinoa is cooked and liquid is absorbed.
2. Heat olive oil in a skillet over medium heat. Add diced onion and minced garlic, and sauté until softened and fragrant.
3. Add diced carrot and diced bell pepper to the skillet. Cook until vegetables are tender.
4. Stir cooked quinoa and frozen peas into the skillet. Cook for an additional 2-3 minutes, or until peas are heated through.
5. Season with salt and pepper to taste.
6. Garnish with fresh parsley before serving.

Per serving
Calories: 100| Carbs: 16g| Fats: 3g| Protein: 4g

Balsamic Glazed Roasted Carrots

Time: 30 minutes| Difficulty: Easy| Serving 2

1 pound carrots, peeled and halved lengthwise
2 tablespoons olive oil
2 tablespoons balsamic vinegar
1 tablespoon honey or maple syrup
Salt and pepper to taste
Fresh parsley for garnish

1. Preheat oven to 400°F (200°C).
2. In a small bowl, whisk together olive oil, balsamic vinegar, honey or maple syrup, salt, and pepper.
3. Place halved carrots on a baking sheet lined with parchment paper.
4. Drizzle balsamic glaze over the carrots, tossing to coat evenly.
5. Roast in the preheated oven for 20-25 minutes, or until carrots are tender and caramelized, stirring halfway through.
6. Garnish with fresh parsley before serving.
7. Serve hot.

Per serving
Calories: 60| Carbs: 8g| Fats: 3g| Protein: 1g

Lemon Herb Quinoa Salad

Time: 25 minutes| Difficulty: Easy| Serving 2

1 cup quinoa
2 cups vegetable broth
1 lemon, juiced and zest
2 tablespoons olive oil
1/4 cup chopped fresh parsley
1/4 cup chopped fresh mint
Salt and pepper to taste

1. Rinse quinoa under cold water, then combine with vegetable broth in a saucepan. Bring to a boil, then reduce heat to low, cover, and simmer for 15-20 minutes, or until quinoa is cooked and liquid is absorbed.
2. In a small bowl, whisk together lemon juice, lemon zest, olive oil, chopped fresh parsley, and chopped fresh mint.
3. Transfer cooked quinoa to a large bowl. Pour the lemon herb dressing over the quinoa and toss until evenly coated.
4. Season with salt and pepper to taste.
5. Serve chilled or at room temperature.

Per serving: Calories: 100| Carbs: 16g| Fats: 4g| Protein: 3g

Garlic Mashed Cauliflower

Time: 25 minutes| Difficulty: Easy| Serving 2

1 head cauliflower, chopped into florets
2 cloves garlic, minced
2 tablespoons olive oil
Salt and pepper to taste
Fresh chives for garnish (optional)

1. Steam cauliflower florets until tender, about 10-12 minutes.
2. Heat olive oil in a skillet over medium heat. Add minced garlic and sauté until fragrant, about 1-2 minutes.
3. Transfer steamed cauliflower to a food processor. Add sautéed garlic, olive oil, salt, and pepper. Blend until smooth and creamy.
4. Adjust seasoning to taste.
5. Garnish with fresh chives if desired.
6. Serve hot.

Per serving: Calories: 40| Carbs: 4g| Fats: 3g| Protein: 2g

Roasted Brussels Sprouts

Time: 30 minutes| Difficulty: Easy| Serving 2

1 pound Brussels sprouts, trimmed and halved
2 tablespoons olive oil
Salt and pepper to taste

1. Preheat oven to 400°F (200°C).
2. Toss Brussels sprouts with olive oil, salt, and pepper in a bowl until evenly coated.
3. Spread Brussels sprouts in a single layer on a baking sheet.
4. Roast in the preheated oven for 20-25 minutes, or until Brussels sprouts are tender and caramelized, stirring halfway through.
5. Serve hot.

Per serving
Calories: 50| Carbs: 6g| Fats: 3g| Protein: 2g

Lemon Garlic Roasted Broccoli

Time: 20 minutes| Difficulty: Easy| Serving 2

1 pound broccoli florets
2 tablespoons olive oil
2 cloves garlic, minced
1 lemon juiced and zest
Salt and pepper to taste

1. Preheat oven to 425°F (220°C).
2. Toss broccoli florets with olive oil, minced garlic, lemon juice, lemon zest, salt, and pepper in a bowl until evenly coated.
3. Spread broccoli florets in a single layer on a baking sheet lined with parchment paper.
4. Roast in the preheated oven for 15-20 minutes, or until broccoli is tender and slightly browned, stirring halfway through.
5. Serve hot.

Per serving
Calories: 40| Carbs: 6g| Fats: 2g| Protein: 2g

Steamed Asparagus

Time: 15 minutes| Difficulty: Easy| Serving 2

1 bunch asparagus, trimmed
Salt and pepper to taste
Lemon wedges for serving (optional)

1. Bring a pot of water to a boil.
2. Place trimmed asparagus in a steamer basket over the boiling water. Cover and steam for 5-7 minutes, or until asparagus is tender-crisp.
3. Season with salt and pepper to taste.
4. Serve hot with lemon wedges if desired.

Per serving
Calories: 20| Carbs: 4g| Fats: 0g| Protein: 2g

Grilled Portobello Mushroom Caps

Time: 20 minutes| Difficulty: Easy| Serving 2

4 large Portobello mushroom caps
2 tablespoons balsamic vinegar
2 tablespoons olive oil
2 cloves garlic, minced
Salt and pepper to taste
Fresh parsley for garnish

1. Preheat grill or grill pan to medium-high heat.
2. In a small bowl, whisk together balsamic vinegar, olive oil, minced garlic, salt, and pepper.
3. Brush both sides of Portobello mushroom caps with the balsamic mixture.
4. Grill mushroom caps for 5-7 minutes on each side, or until tender and grill marks appear.
5. Garnish with fresh parsley before serving.
6. Serve hot.

Per serving
Calories: 40| Carbs: 3g| Fats: 3g| Protein: 2g

Garlic Roasted Cauliflower

Time: 25 minutes| Difficulty: Easy| Serving 2

1 head cauliflower, chopped into florets
2 tablespoons olive oil
2 cloves garlic, minced

1. Preheat oven to 425°F (220°C).
2. Toss cauliflower florets with olive oil, minced garlic, salt, and pepper in a bowl until evenly coated.
3. Spread cauliflower florets in a single layer on a baking sheet lined with parchment paper.
4. Roast in the preheated oven for 20-25 minutes, or until cauliflower is tender and caramelized, stirring halfway through.

Per serving
Calories: 40| Carbs: 6g| Fats: 2g| Protein: 2g

Baked Sweet Potato Fries

Time: 30 minutes| Difficulty: Easy| Serving 2

2 large sweet potatoes cut into fries
2 tablespoons olive oil
1 teaspoon paprika
1/2 teaspoon garlic powder

1. Preheat oven to 425°F (220°C).
2. In a large bowl, toss sweet potato fries with olive oil, paprika, garlic powder, salt, and pepper until evenly coated.
3. Spread sweet potato fries in a single layer on a baking sheet lined with parchment paper.
4. Bake in the preheated oven for 25-30 minutes, or until fries are crispy and golden brown, flipping halfway through.

Per serving : Calories: 50| Carbohydrates: 8g| Fats: 2g| Protein: 1g

Steamed Green Beans with Almonds

Time: 20 minutes| Difficulty: Easy| Serving 2

1 pound green beans, trimmed
2 tablespoons sliced almonds
1 tablespoon olive oil
Salt and pepper to taste
Lemon wedges for serving (optional)

1. Bring a pot of water to a boil.
2. Place trimmed green beans in a steamer basket over the boiling water. Cover and steam for 5-7 minutes, or until green beans are tender-crisp.
3. While the green beans are steaming, heat olive oil in a skillet over medium heat. Add sliced almonds and toast until golden brown and fragrant, about 2-3 minutes.
4. Transfer steamed green beans to a serving dish. Drizzle with toasted almond slices.
5. Season with salt and pepper to taste.
6. Serve hot with lemon wedges if desired.

Per serving
Calories: 50| Carbs: 6g| Fats: 3g| Protein: 2g

Sauteed Spinach with Garlic and Lemon

Time: 15 minutes| Difficulty: Easy| Serving 2

8 ounces baby spinach
2 cloves garlic, minced
1 tablespoon olive oil
1 lemon juiced and zest

1. Heat olive oil in a large skillet over medium heat. Add minced garlic and sauté until fragrant, about 1-2 minutes.
2. Add baby spinach to the skillet in batches, tossing until wilted.
3. Once all the spinach is wilted, add lemon juice and zest to the skillet. Stir well to combine.

Per serving: Calories: 20| Carbs: 2g| Fats: 1g| Protein: 2g

Herb Roasted Potatoes

Time: 40 minutes| Difficulty: Easy| Serving 2

1 pound baby potatoes, halved
2 tablespoons olive oil
2 cloves garlic, minced
1 teaspoon dried rosemary
1 teaspoon dried thyme

1. Preheat oven to 400°F (200°C).
2. Toss halved baby potatoes with olive oil, minced garlic, dried rosemary, dried thyme, salt, and pepper in a bowl until evenly coated.
3. Spread potatoes in a single layer on a baking sheet lined with parchment paper.
4. Roast in the preheated oven for 30-35 minutes, or until potatoes are golden brown and crispy, stirring halfway through.

Per serving: Calories: 60| Carbs: 10g| Fats: 3g| Protein: 1g

Grilled Eggplant Slices

Time: 20 minutes| Difficulty: Easy| Serving 2

1 large eggplant, sliced into rounds
2 tablespoons olive oil
1 teaspoon dried oregano
1 teaspoon dried thyme
Salt and pepper to taste

1. Preheat grill or grill pan to medium-high heat.
2. Brush eggplant slices with olive oil on both sides.
3. Sprinkle dried oregano, dried thyme, salt, and pepper on both sides of eggplant slices.
4. Grill eggplant slices for 3-4 minutes on each side, or until tender and grill marks appear.
5. Serve hot.

Per serving
Calories: 40| Carbs: 6g| Fats: 2g| Protein: 1g

Roasted Beet Salad with Goat Cheese and Walnuts

Time: 50 minutes| Difficulty: Intermediate| Serving 2

2 large beets, peeled and diced
2 tablespoons olive oil
Salt and pepper to taste
2 cups mixed greens
1/4 cup crumbled goat cheese
1/4 cup chopped walnuts
Balsamic glaze for drizzling

1. Preheat oven to 400°F (200°C).
2. Toss diced beets with olive oil, salt, and pepper in a bowl until evenly coated.
3. Spread beets in a single layer on a baking sheet lined with parchment paper.
4. Roast in the preheated oven for 40-45 minutes, or until beets are tender and caramelized, stirring halfway through.
5. In a serving bowl, arrange mixed greens. Top with roasted beets, crumbled goat cheese, and chopped walnuts.
6. Drizzle balsamic glaze over the salad before serving.
7. Serve warm or at room temperature.

Per serving:
Calories: 70| Carbs: 6g| Fats: 5g| Protein: 2g

Oven-Roasted Tomatoes

Time: 35 minutes| Difficulty: Easy| Serving 2

1 pound cherry tomatoes
2 tablespoons olive oil
2 cloves garlic, minced
1 teaspoon dried basil
Salt and pepper to taste
Fresh basil for garnish

1. Preheat oven to 375°F (190°C).
2. Toss cherry tomatoes with olive oil, minced garlic, dried basil, salt, and pepper in a bowl until evenly coated.
3. Spread cherry tomatoes in a single layer on a baking sheet lined with parchment paper.
4. Roast in the preheated oven for 25-30 minutes, or until tomatoes are soft and caramelized, stirring halfway through.
5. Garnish with fresh basil before serving.
6. Serve hot or at room temperature.

Per serving
Calories: 40| Carbohydrates: 4g| Fats: 3g| Protein: 1g

Sauteed Mushrooms with Garlic and Herbs

Time: 20 minutes| Difficulty: Easy| Serving 2

8 ounces mushrooms, sliced
2 cloves garlic, minced
2 tablespoons olive oil
1 tablespoon chopped fresh parsley
1 tablespoon chopped fresh thyme
Salt and pepper to taste

1. Heat olive oil in a large skillet over medium heat. Add minced garlic and sauté until fragrant, about 1-2 minutes.
2. Add sliced mushrooms to the skillet. Cook until mushrooms are tender and golden brown, stirring occasionally.
3. Stir in chopped fresh parsley and chopped fresh thyme. Cook for an additional 1-2 minutes.
4. Season with salt and pepper to taste.
5. Serve hot.

Per serving
Calories: 30| Carbs: 2g| Fats: 3g| Protein: 1g

Herbed Roasted Carrots and Parsnips

Time: 30 minutes| Difficulty: Easy| Serving 2

1 pound carrots, peeled and cut into sticks
1 pound parsnips, peeled and cut into sticks
2 tablespoons olive oil
1 tablespoon chopped fresh rosemary
1 tablespoon chopped fresh thyme
Salt and pepper to taste

1. Preheat oven to 400°F (200°C).
2. Toss carrot sticks and parsnip sticks with olive oil, chopped fresh rosemary, chopped fresh thyme, salt, and pepper in a bowl until evenly coated.
3. Spread carrot and parsnip sticks in a single layer on a baking sheet lined with parchment paper.
4. Roast in the preheated oven for 25-30 minutes, or until vegetables are tender and caramelized, stirring halfway through.
5. Serve hot.

Per serving
Calories: 60| Carbs: 8g| Fats: 3g| Protein: 1g

Roasted Brussels Sprouts with Balsamic Glaze

Time: 30 minutes| Difficulty: Easy| Serving 2

1 pound Brussels sprouts, trimmed and halved
2 tablespoons olive oil
Salt and pepper to taste
2 tablespoons balsamic glaze

1. Preheat oven to 400°F (200°C).
2. Toss halved Brussels sprouts with olive oil, salt, and pepper in a bowl until evenly coated.
3. Spread Brussels sprouts in a single layer on a baking sheet lined with parchment paper.
4. Roast in the preheated oven for 25-30 minutes, or until Brussels sprouts are tender and caramelized, stirring halfway through.
5. Drizzle roasted Brussels sprouts with balsamic glaze before serving.
6. Serve hot.

Per serving:
Calories: 50| Carbs: 6g| Fats: 3g| Protein: 2g

Garlic Herb Roasted Potatoes

Time: 35 minutes| Difficulty: Easy| Serving 2

1 pound baby potatoes, halved
2 tablespoons olive oil
2 cloves garlic, minced
1 tablespoon chopped fresh rosemary
1 tablespoon chopped fresh thyme
Salt and pepper to taste

1. Preheat oven to 425°F (220°C).
2. Toss halved baby potatoes with olive oil, minced garlic, chopped fresh rosemary, chopped fresh thyme, salt, and pepper in a bowl until evenly coated.
3. Spread potatoes in a single layer on a baking sheet lined with parchment paper.
4. Roast in the preheated oven for 30-35 minutes, or until potatoes are golden brown and crispy, stirring halfway through.
5. Serve hot.

Per serving
Calories: 60| Carbs: 10g| Fats: 3g| Protein: 1g

Sauteed Kale with Garlic and Lemon

Time: 15 minutes| Difficulty: Easy| Serving 2

1 bunch kale, stems removed and leaves chopped
2 cloves garlic, minced
2 tablespoons olive oil
1 lemon juiced and zest
Salt and pepper to taste

1. Heat olive oil in a large skillet over medium heat. Add minced garlic and sauté until fragrant, about 1-2 minutes.
2. Add chopped kale to the skillet. Cook until kale is wilted and tender, stirring occasionally.
3. Once the kale is cooked, add lemon juice and zest to the skillet. Stir well to combine.
4. Season with salt and pepper to taste.
5. Serve hot.

Per serving: Calories: 30| Carbs: 4g| Fats: 2g| Protein: 2g

Grilled Asparagus with Lemon and Parmesan

Time: 15 minutes| Difficulty: Easy| Serving 2

1 pound asparagus, trimmed
2 tablespoons olive oil
1 lemon, juiced and zest
1/4 cup grated Parmesan cheese
Salt and pepper to taste

1. Preheat grill or grill pan to medium-high heat.
2. Toss trimmed asparagus with olive oil, lemon juice, lemon zest, salt, and pepper in a bowl until evenly coated.
3. Grill asparagus spears for 3-4 minutes on each side, or until tender and grill marks appear.
4. Transfer grilled asparagus to a serving platter. Sprinkle grated Parmesan cheese on top.
5. Serve hot.

Per serving:: Calories: 50| Carbs: 4g| Fats: 4g| Protein: 3g

Roasted Butternut Squash with Cinnamon

Time: 40 minutes| Difficulty: Easy| Serving 2

1 medium butternut squash, peeled, seeded, and cut into cubes
2 tablespoons olive oil
1 teaspoon ground cinnamon
Salt and pepper to taste

1. Preheat oven to 400°F (200°C).
2. Toss butternut squash cubes with olive oil, ground cinnamon, salt, and pepper in a bowl until evenly coated.
3. Spread butternut squash cubes in a single layer on a baking sheet lined with parchment paper.
4. Roast in the preheated oven for 30-35 minutes, or until squash is tender and caramelized, stirring halfway through.
5. Serve hot.

Per serving
Calories: 60| Carbs: 10g| Fats: 3g| Protein: 1g

Roasted Chickpeas

Time: 40 minutes| Difficulty: Easy| Serving 2

1 can (15 ounces) chickpeas, drained and rinsed
1 tablespoon olive oil
1 teaspoon ground cumin and 1 teaspoon paprika
1/2 teaspoon garlic powder

1. Preheat oven to 400°F (200°C).
2. Pat chickpeas dry with paper towels to remove excess moisture.
3. In a bowl, toss chickpeas with olive oil, ground cumin, paprika, garlic powder, salt, and pepper until evenly coated.
4. Spread chickpeas in a single layer on a baking sheet lined with parchment paper.
5. Roast in the preheated oven for 30-35 minutes, or until chickpeas are crispy, stirring halfway through.
6. Allow roasted chickpeas to cool before serving.

Per serving: Calories: 60| Carbs: 10g| Fats: 2g| Protein: 3g

Caprese Skewers with Balsamic Glaze

Time: 15 minutes| Difficulty: Easy| Serving 2

Cherry tomatoes and Fresh basil leaves
Fresh mozzarella balls
Balsamic glaze

1. Thread one cherry tomato, one mozzarella-ball, and one fresh basil leaf onto each skewer.
2. Arrange the skewers on a serving platter.
3. Drizzle with balsamic glaze just before serving.

Per serving: Calories: 30| Carbs: 2g| Fats: 2g| Protein: 2g

Stuffed Mini Bell Peppers

Time: 20 minutes| Difficulty: Easy| Serving 2

Mini bell peppers, halved and seeds removed
Hummus
Cherry tomatoes, halved
Fresh parsley, chopped

1. Fill each mini bell pepper half with a spoonful of hummus.
2. Top with a halved cherry tomato.
3. Garnish with chopped fresh parsley.
4. Serve chilled or at room temperature.

Per serving (2 stuffed pepper halves)
Calories: 50| Carbs: 6g| Fats: 2g| Protein: 2g

Avocado Hummus with Whole Wheat Pita Chips

Time: 15 minutes| Difficulty: Easy| Serving 2

1 ripe avocado, peeled and pitted
1 can (15 ounces) chickpeas, drained and rinsed
2 tablespoons tahini
2 tablespoons lemon juice
1 clove garlic, minced
2 tablespoons olive oil
Salt and pepper to taste
Whole wheat pita bread, cut into wedges and toasted

1. In a food processor, combine ripe avocado, chickpeas, tahini, lemon juice, minced garlic, olive oil, salt, and pepper.
2. Blend until smooth and creamy.
3. Serve the avocado hummus with toasted whole wheat pita wedges for dipping.

Per serving
Calories: 80| Carbs: 10g| Fats: 4g| Protein: 3g

Cauliflower Buffalo Bites

Time: 30 minutes| Difficulty: Intermediate| Serving 2

1 head cauliflower, cut into florets
1/2 cup buffalo sauce
1 tablespoon melted butter or olive oil
1/2 teaspoon garlic powder
Ranch or blue cheese dressing for dipping

1. Preheat oven to 425°F (220°C). Line a baking sheet with parchment paper.
2. In a bowl, whisk together buffalo sauce, melted butter or olive oil, and garlic powder.
3. Toss cauliflower florets in the buffalo sauce mixture until evenly coated.
4. Spread coated cauliflower florets in a single layer on the prepared baking sheet.
5. Bake for 20-25 minutes, or until cauliflower is tender and edges are crispy.
6. Serve hot with ranch or blue cheese dressing for dipping.

Per serving: Calories: 50| Carbs: 5g| Fats: 3g| Protein: 2g

Mediterranean Stuffed Dates

Time: 10 minutes| Difficulty: Easy| Serving 2

Medjool dates, pitted
Soft goat cheese
Walnut halves

1. Stuff each pitted date with a small amount of soft goat cheese.
2. Press a walnut half on top of the goat cheese.
3. Arrange stuffed dates on a serving platter.

Per serving (2 stuffed dates)
Calories: 80| Carbs: 12g| Fats: 3g| Protein: 2g

Guacamole Stuffed Mini Peppers

Time: 15 minutes| Difficulty: Easy| Serving 2

Mini sweet peppers, halved and seeded
Ripe avocado, mashed
Cherry tomatoes, diced
Red onion, finely chopped
Jalapeño, seeded and minced (optional)
Lime juice
Salt and pepper to taste
Fresh cilantro for garnish

1. In a bowl, combine mashed avocado, diced cherry tomatoes, finely chopped red onion, minced jalapeño (if using), lime juice, salt, and pepper.
2. Fill each mini pepper half with the guacamole mixture.
3. Garnish with fresh cilantro before serving.

Per serving: (2 stuffed mini peppers): Calories:60| Carbs: 4g| Fats: 4g| Protein: 2g

Smoked Salmon Cucumber Bites

Time: 10 minutes| Difficulty: Easy| Serving 2

English cucumber, sliced into rounds
Smoked salmon slices
Cream cheese
Fresh dill for garnish

1. Spread a thin layer of cream cheese on each cucumber round.
2. Top with a piece of smoked salmon.
3. Garnish with fresh dill before serving.

Per serving (2 cucumber bites): Calories: 40| Carbs: 2g| Fats: 3g| Protein: 3g

Greek Yogurt Dip with Veggies

Time: 10 minutes| Difficulty: Easy| Serving 2

1 cup Greek yogurt
1 tablespoon lemon juice
1 clove garlic, minced
1 tablespoon chopped fresh dill
Salt and pepper to taste
Assorted vegetables for dipping (carrots, cucumber, bell peppers, etc.)

1. In a mixing bowl, combine Greek yogurt, lemon juice, minced garlic, chopped fresh dill, salt, and pepper.
2. Stir until well combined.
3. Serve the yogurt dip with assorted vegetables for dipping.

Per serving
Calories: 50| Carbs: 4g| Fats: 1g| Protein: 6g

Cucumber Slices with Herbed Cream Cheese

Time: 10 minutes| Difficulty: Easy| Serving 2

English cucumber, sliced into rounds
Cream cheese
Fresh herbs (dill, chives, parsley, etc.)
Salt and pepper to taste

1. Spread a thin layer of cream cheese on each cucumber round.
2. Sprinkle with chopped fresh herbs.
3. Season with salt and pepper to taste.
4. Serve chilled.

Per serving
Calories: 50| Carbs: 2g| Fats: 4g| Protein: 2g

Apple Slices with Low-Fat Cheese

Time: 5 minutes| Difficulty: Easy| Serving 2

1 medium apple, sliced
2 slices of low-fat cheese (such as mozzarella or cheddar)

1. Wash and slice the apple into thin slices.
2. Cut the low-fat cheese slices into smaller pieces or strips.
3. Arrange the apple slices and cheese on a plate or in a portable container.
4. Serve and enjoy as a simple and satisfying snack.

Per serving
Calories: 120| Protein: 6g| Carbs: 15g| Fat: 4g| Fiber: 3g

Baked Zucchini Fries

Time: 30 minutes| Difficulty: Intermediate| Serving 2

2 medium zucchinis cut into fries
1/2 cup breadcrumbs
1/4 cup grated Parmesan cheese
1 teaspoon Italian seasoning
Salt and pepper to taste
1 egg, beaten
Cooking spray

1. Preheat oven to 425°F (220°C). Line a baking sheet with parchment paper and lightly coat with cooking spray.
2. In a shallow dish, combine breadcrumbs, Parmesan cheese, Italian seasoning, salt, and pepper.
3. Dip zucchini fries into beaten egg, then coat with breadcrumb mixture.
4. Place coated zucchini fries on the prepared baking sheet in a single layer.
5. Bake for 20-25 minutes, or until golden brown and crispy.
6. Serve hot with your favorite dipping sauce.

Per serving (6 zucchini fries)
Calories: 70| Carbs: 10g| Fats: 2g| Protein: 4g

Cucumber Avocado Rolls

Time: 15 minutes| Difficulty: Easy| Serving 2

English cucumber
Avocado
Red bell pepper, thinly sliced
Carrot, thinly sliced
Alfalfa sprouts
Hummus
Sesame seeds for garnish (optional)

1. Using a vegetable peeler, slice the cucumber lengthwise into thin strips.
2. Spread a thin layer of hummus on each cucumber strip.
3. Place a few slices of avocado, red bell pepper, carrot, and a small handful of alfalfa sprouts at one end of the cucumber strip.
4. Roll up the cucumbers strip tightly, enclosing the filling.
5. Secure with a toothpick if necessary.
6. Sprinkle with sesame seeds for garnish if desired.
7. Serve chilled.

Per serving (2 cucumber rolls)
Calories: 60| Carbs: 5g| Fats: 4g| Protein: 2g

Quinoa and Black Bean Stuffed Mushrooms

Time: 30 minutes| Difficulty: Intermediate| Serving 2

Large mushrooms, stems removed
Cooked quinoa
Black beans, drained and rinsed
Salsa
Shredded cheese (optional)
Fresh cilantro for garnish

1. Preheat oven to 375°F (190°C). Line a baking sheet with parchment paper.
2. In a bowl, combine cooked quinoa, black beans, and salsa.
3. Stuff each mushroom cap with the quinoa and black bean mixture.
4. If desired, sprinkle shredded cheese on top of each stuffed mushroom.
5. Place stuffed mushrooms on the prepared baking sheet.
6. Bake for 20-25 minutes, or until mushrooms are tender and filling is heated through.
7. Garnish with fresh cilantro before serving.

Per serving (2 stuffed mushrooms)
Calories: 70| Carbs: 10g|Fats: 2g| Protein: 4g

Hummus with Veggie Sticks

Time: 15 minutes| Difficulty: Easy| Serving 2

1 cup shelled hummus, cooked and cooled
1 tablespoon tahini
2 cloves garlic, minced
2 tablespoons lemon juice
2 tablespoons olive oil
Salt and pepper to taste
Assorted veggie sticks (carrots, celery, bell peppers, etc.) for dipping

1. In a food processor, combine cooked hummus, tahini, minced garlic, lemon juice, olive oil, salt, and pepper.
2. Blend until smooth and creamy, adding water as needed to reach desired consistency.
3. Transfer hummus to a serving bowl.
4. Serve with assorted veggie sticks for dipping.

Per serving (2 tablespoons hummus with veggies): Calories: 50| Carbs: 4g| Fats: 3g| Protein: 3g

Spinach and Artichoke Dip with Whole Wheat Pita Chips

Time: 30 minutes| Difficulty: Intermediate | Serving 2

1 cup frozen chopped spinach, thawed and drained
1 can (14 ounces) artichoke hearts, drained and chopped
1/2 cup plain Greek yogurt
1/4 cup grated Parmesan cheese
1/4 cup shredded mozzarella cheese
1/4 teaspoon garlic powder
Salt and pepper to taste
Whole wheat pita bread, cut into wedges and toasted

1. Preheat oven to 375°F (190°C).
2. In a mixing bowl, combine chopped spinach, chopped artichoke hearts, Greek yogurt, grated Parmesan cheese, shredded mozzarella cheese, garlic powder, salt, and pepper.
3. Transfer the mixture to a baking dish.
4. Bake for 20-25 minutes, or until bubbly and golden brown on top.
5. Serve hot with whole wheat pita chips for dipping

Per serving (2 tablespoons dip with pita chips): Calories: 80| Carbs: 10g| Fats: 3g| Protein: 5g

Trail Mix

Time: 5 minutes| Difficulty: Easy| Serving 2

1/2 cup almonds
1/2 cup cashews
1/4 cup dried cranberries
1/4 cup pumpkin seeds
1/4 cup dark chocolate chips (optional)

1. In a mixing bowl, combine all the ingredients.
2. Toss gently to mix evenly.
3. Divide the trail mix into two servings and transfer to portable containers.
4. Enjoy as a convenient and energizing snack on the go.

Per serving: Calories: 300| Protein: 8g| Carbs: 20g| Fat: 20g| Fiber: 5g

Avocado Cucumber Rolls

Time: 15 minutes| Difficulty: Easy| Serving 2

English cucumber
Avocado
Red bell pepper, thinly sliced
Carrot, thinly sliced
Alfalfa sprouts
Hummus
Sesame seeds for garnish (optional)

1. Using a vegetable peeler, slice the cucumber lengthwise into thin strips.
2. Spread a thin layer of hummus on each cucumber strip.
3. Place a few slices of avocado, red bell pepper, carrot, and a small handful of alfalfa sprouts at one end of the cucumber strip.
4. Roll up the cucumber strips tightly, enclosing the filling.
5. Secure with a toothpick if necessary.
6. Sprinkle with sesame seeds for garnish if desired.
7. Serve chilled.

Per serving (2 cucumber rolls): Calories: 60| Carbs: 5g| Fats: 4g| Protein: 2g

Greek Yogurt with Berries and Almonds

Time: 5 minutes| Difficulty: Easy| Serving 2

1 cup Greek yogurt
1/2 cup mixed berries (such as strawberries, blueberries, and raspberries)
1/4 cup almonds, sliced or chopped

1. In serving bowls or jars, divide the Greek yogurt evenly.
2. Top each portion of Greek yogurt with mixed berries and almonds.
3. Serve immediately or store in the refrigerator until ready to eat.

Per serving : Calories: 200| Protein: 15g| Carbs: 15g| Fat: 10g\ Fiber: 4g

Banana Slices with Almond Butter

Time: 5 minutes| Difficulty: Easy| Serving 2

1 banana, sliced
2 tablespoons almond butter

1. Spread almond butter on banana slices.
2. Arrange the banana slices on a plate or in a portable container.
3. Serve immediately for a delicious and satisfying snack.

Per serving : Calories: 220| Protein: 5g| Carbs: 25g| Fat: 12g| Fiber: 4g

Cherry Tomatoes with Cottage Cheese

Time: 5 minutes| Difficulty: Easy| Serving 2

1 cup cherry tomatoes
1/2 cup cottage cheese

1. Wash the cherry tomatoes and place them in a bowl.
2. Serve the cherry tomatoes with cottage cheese on the side.
3. Enjoy this refreshing and protein-rich snack option.

Per serving
Calories: 120| Protein: 10g| Carbs: 10g| Fat: 4g| Fiber: 2g

2.8 Desserts Recipes

Whole Wheat Banana Pancakes

Time: 15 minutes| Difficulty: Easy| Serving 2

1 ripe banana, mashed
2 eggs
1/2 cup whole wheat flour
1/4 cup almond milk
1/2 teaspoon baking powder
1/4 teaspoon cinnamon
1/4 teaspoon vanilla extract
Butter or oil for cooking

1. In a mixing bowl, whisk together mashed banana, eggs, whole wheat flour, almond milk, baking powder, cinnamon, and vanilla extract until smooth.
2. Heat a non-stick skillet over medium heat and add butter or oil.
3. Pour pancake batter onto the skillet to form small pancakes.
4. Cook for 2-3 minutes on each side, until golden brown and cooked through.
5. Serve warm with your favorite toppings, such as sliced fruit or a drizzle of honey.

Per serving : Calories: 250| Protein: 10g| Carbs: 30g| Fat: 10g| Fiber: 4g

Almond Flour Pancakes

Time: 15 minutes| Difficulty: Easy| Serving 2
1 cup almond flour and 1/4 cup almond milk
2 eggs
1 tablespoon honey (optional)
1/2 teaspoon baking powder
Pinch of salt and Oil for cooking

1. In a mixing bowl, whisk almond flour, eggs, almond milk, honey (if using), baking powder, and salt until well combined.
2. Heat a non-stick skillet over medium heat and add oil.
3. Pour pancake batter onto the skillet to form small pancakes.
4. Cook for 2-3 minutes on each side, until golden brown and cooked through.
5. Serve warm with your favorite toppings, such as fresh berries or a drizzle of honey.

Per serving : Calories: 250| Protein: 8g| Carbs: 15g| Fat: 18g| Fiber: 3g

Mixed Berry Parfait

Time: 10 minutes| Difficulty: Easy| Serving 2

1 cup Greek yogurt (unsweetened)
1 cup mixed berries (strawberries, blueberries, raspberries)
2 tablespoons granola and 1 tablespoon honey (optional)

1. In two serving glasses, layer Greek yogurt, mixed berries, and granola (if using), repeating until glasses are filled.
2. Drizzle honey or maple syrup over the top if desired.

Per serving: Calories: 120| Carbs: 15g| Fats: 3g| Protein: 10g

Whole Wheat Banana Bread

Time: 1 hour| Difficulty: Moderate| Serving 2

2 ripe bananas, mashed
1/4 cup honey or maple syrup
1/4 cup olive oil
2 eggs
1 teaspoon vanilla extract
1 1/2 cups whole wheat flour
1 teaspoon baking powder
1/2 teaspoon baking soda
1/2 teaspoon cinnamon
Pinch of salt
Chopped nuts or chocolate chips for topping (optional)

1. Preheat the oven to 350°F (175°C) and grease a loaf pan with olive oil.
2. In a mixing bowl, whisk together mashed bananas, honey or maple syrup, olive oil, eggs, and vanilla extract until well combined.
3. In a separate bowl, combine whole wheat flour, baking powder, baking soda, cinnamon, and salt.
4. Gradually add the dry ingredients to the wet ingredients, stirring until just combined.
5. Pour the batter into the prepared loaf pan and smooth the top with a spatula.
6. If desired, sprinkle chopped nuts or chocolate chips over the top of the batter.
7. Bake for 45-50 minutes, or until a toothpick inserted into the center comes out clean.
8. Allow the banana bread to cool in the pan for 10 minutes before transferring it to a wire rack to cool completely.
9. Slice and serve warm or at room temperature.

Per serving
Calories: 200| Protein: 6g| Carbs: 30g|Fat: 7g| Fiber: 4g

Mediterranean Egg Muffins

Time: 20 minutes| Difficulty: Easy| Serving 2

6 large eggs
1/2 cup chopped spinach
1/4 cup diced tomatoes
1/4 cup crumbled feta cheese
2 tablespoons chopped olives
Salt and pepper to taste
Olive oil for greasing muffin tin

1. Preheat the oven to 350°F (175°C) and grease a muffin tin with olive oil.
2. In a mixing bowl, whisk together eggs, salt, and pepper until well beaten.
3. Stir in chopped spinach, diced tomatoes, crumbled feta cheese, and chopped olives.
4. Pour the egg mixture into the prepared muffin tin, filling each cup about two-thirds full.
5. Bake for 15-20 minutes, or until the egg muffins are set and golden brown on top.
6. Remove from the oven and let them cool slightly before serving.
7. Serve warm or at room temperature, and enjoy these protein-packed egg muffins!

Per serving
Calories: 180| Protein: 12g| Carbs: 4g| Fat: 12g| Fiber: 2g

Lemon Coconut Bliss Balls

Time: 15 minutes (plus chilling time)| Difficulty: Easy| for 2

1/2 cup raw cashews
1/2 cup unsweetened shredded coconut
2 tablespoons coconut oil, melted
Zest and juice of 1 lemon
1 tablespoon maple syrup or honey
Pinch of salt

1. In a food processor, combine raw cashews, shredded coconut, melted coconut oil, lemon zest, lemon juice, maple syrup or honey, and a pinch of salt.
2. Process until mixture comes together and forms dough.
3. Roll the dough into small balls.
4. Place bliss balls on a plate and chill in the refrigerator for at least 30 minutes before serving.

Per serving (2 bliss balls): Calories: 120|Carbs: 7g| Fats: 10g| Protein: 2g

Banana Oatmeal Muffins

Time: 25 minutes| Difficulty: Easy| Serving 2

2 ripe bananas, mashed
1 cup rolled oats
1/4 cup almond flour
2 eggs
1/4 cup honey or maple syrup
1 teaspoon baking powder
1/2 teaspoon cinnamon
Pinch of salt

1. Preheat the oven to 350°F (175°C) and line a muffin tin with paper liners.
2. In a large mixing bowl, combine mashed bananas, rolled oats, almond flour, eggs, honey or maple syrup, baking powder, cinnamon, and salt. Mix until well combined.
3. Spoon the batter into the prepared muffin tin, filling each cup about two-thirds full.
4. Bake for 20-25 minutes, until the muffins are golden brown and a toothpick inserted into the center comes out clean.
5. Allow the muffins to cool in the tin for 5 minutes, and then transfer to a wire rack to cool completely.

Per serving : Calories: 200| Protein: 6g| Carbs: 30g| Fat: 7g| Fiber: 4g

Coconut Mango Popsicles

Time: 10 minutes (plus freezing time)| Difficulty: Easy| For 2

1 ripe mango, peeled and diced
1/2 cup coconut milk (canned or homemade)
1 tablespoon maple syrup or honey
Unsweetened shredded coconut for topping (optional)

1. In a blender, combine diced mango, coconut milk, and maple syrup or honey.
2. Blend until smooth.
3. Pour the mixture into popsicle molds.
4. Insert popsicle sticks and freeze for at least 4 hours or until firm.
5. Before serving, sprinkle with shredded coconut if desired.

Per serving (1 popsicle): Calories: Approximately 70| Carbs: 10g| Fats: 4g| Protein: 1g

Zucchini and Carrot Breakfast Muffins

Time: 25 minutes| Difficulty: Easy| Serving 2

1 cup grated zucchini
1 cup grated carrot
1/4 cup chopped nuts (such as walnuts or pecans)
1/4 cup raisins or dried cranberries
2 eggs
1/4 cup honey or maple syrup
1/4 cup olive oil
1 teaspoon vanilla extract
1 cup whole wheat flour
1 teaspoon baking powder
1/2 teaspoon baking soda
1/2 teaspoon cinnamon

1. Preheat the oven to 350°F (175°C) and line a muffin tin with paper liners.
2. In a mixing bowl, combine grated zucchini, grated carrot, chopped nuts, and raisins or dried cranberries.
3. In a separate bowl, whisk together eggs, honey or maple syrup, olive oil, and vanilla extract.
4. Gradually add the wet ingredients to the dry ingredients, stirring until just combined.
5. Spoon the batter into the prepared muffin tin, filling each cup about two-thirds full.
6. Bake for 20-25 minutes, or until the muffins are golden brown and a toothpick inserted into the center comes out clean.
7. Allow the muffins to cool in the tin for 5 minutes before transferring them to a wire rack to cool completely.

Per serving
Calories: 220|Protein: 6g| Carbs: 30g| Fat: 10g| Fiber: 5g

Banana Oat Cookies

Time: 20 minutes| Difficulty: Easy| Serving 2

1 ripe banana, mashed
1 cup rolled oats
2 tablespoons almond butter
1 tablespoon maple syrup or honey
1/2 teaspoon vanilla extract
Pinch of cinnamon (optional)

1. Preheat oven to 350°F (175°C) and line a baking sheet with parchment paper.
2. In a bowl, combine mashed banana, rolled oats, almond butter, maple syrup or honey, vanilla extract, and cinnamon (if using).
3. Drop spoonful of the mixture onto the prepared baking sheet and flatten slightly with the back of a spoon.
4. Bake for 12-15 minutes, or until cookies are golden brown around the edges.
5. Let cool before serving.

Per serving (2 cookies)
Calories: 100| Carbs: 15g| Fats: 3g| Protein: 2g

Coconut Chia Seed Pudding

Time: 10 minutes (plus chilling time)| Difficulty: Easy| For 2

1/4 cup chia seeds
1 cup coconut milk (canned or homemade)
1 tablespoon maple syrup or honey
1/2 teaspoon vanilla extract
Shredded coconut for topping

1. In a bowl, whisk together chia seeds, coconut milk, maple syrup or honey, and vanilla extract.
2. Cover and refrigerate for at least 2 hours or overnight, until the mixture thickens to a pudding-like consistency.
3. Serve topped with shredded coconut.

Per serving
Calories: 130| Carbs: 10g| Fats: 10g| Protein: 3g

Berry Chia Seed Pudding

Time: 10 minutes (plus chilling time)|Difficulty: Easy| For 2

1/4 cup chia seeds
1 cup unsweetened almond milk
1 tablespoon maple syrup or honey
1/2 teaspoon vanilla extract
Mixed berries for topping

1. In a bowl, whisk together chia seeds, almond milk, maple syrup or honey, and vanilla extract.
2. Cover and refrigerate for at least 2 hours or overnight, until the mixture thickens to a pudding-like consistency.
3. Serve topped with mixed berries.

Per serving
Calories: 120| Carbs: 15g| Fats: 5g| Protein: 4g

Baked Apples with Cinnamon

Time: 30 minutes| Difficulty: Easy| Serving 2

2 apples, cored
2 tablespoons almond butter
1 tablespoon maple syrup or honey
1/2 teaspoon cinnamon
Chopped nuts for topping (optional)

1. Preheat oven to 375°F (190°C) and line a baking dish with parchment paper.
2. Place cored apples in the prepared baking dish.
3. In a small bowl, mix together almond butter, maple syrup or honey, and cinnamon.
4. Stuff each apple with the almond butter mixture.
5. Bake for 20-25 minutes, or until apples are tender.
6. Serve hot, sprinkled with chopped nuts if desired.

Per serving
Calories: 150| Carbs: 20g| Fats: 7g| Protein: 2g

Chocolate Avocado Mousse

Time: 15 minutes| Difficulty: Easy| Serving 2

1 ripe avocado
2 tablespoons cocoa powder
2 tablespoons maple syrup or honey
1/2 teaspoon vanilla extract and Pinch of salt
Berries or chopped nuts for topping (optional)

1. Scoop the flesh of the avocado into a blender or food processor.
2. Add cocoa powder, maple syrup or honey, vanilla extract, and a pinch of salt.
3. Blend until smooth and creamy, scraping down the sides as needed.
4. Divide the mousse into serving dishes and chill in the refrigerator for at least 30 minutes.
5. Serve topped with berries or chopped nuts if desired.

Per serving
Calories: 150| Carbs: 15g| Fats: 10g| Protein: 2g

Vanilla Coconut Rice Pudding

Time: 40 minutes| Difficulty: Easy| Serving 2

1/2 cup white rice
2 cups coconut milk (canned or homemade)
1/4 cup maple syrup or honey
1 teaspoon vanilla extract and Pinch of salt
Ground cinnamon for topping (optional)

1. In a saucepan, combine rice, coconut milk, maple syrup or honey, vanilla extract, and a pinch of salt.
2. Bring to a boil, then reduce heat and simmer, stirring occasionally, for 30-35 minutes, or until rice is cooked and mixture thickens.
3. Remove from heat and let cool slightly.
4. Serve warm or chilled, optionally topped with ground cinnamon.

Per serving
Calories: 200| Carbs: 25g| Fats: 10g| Protein: 2g

Cinnamon Baked Pears

Time: 30 minutes| Difficulty: Easy| Serving 2

2 ripe pears, halved and cored, 1 tbs. coconut oil, melted
1 tbs. maple syrup and 1/2 teaspoon cinnamon

1. Preheat oven to 375°F (190°C) and line a baking dish with parchment paper.
2. Place pear halves in the prepared baking dish.
3. In a small bowl, mix together melted coconut oil, maple syrup or honey, and cinnamon.
4. Drizzle the mixture over the pear halves.
5. Bake for 20-25 minutes, or until pears are tender.

Per serving
Calories: 120| Carbs: 20g| Fats: 5g| Protein: 1g

Chocolate Almond Date Balls

Time: 15 min (plus chilling time)| Difficulty: Easy| Serving 2

1/2 cup almonds and 1/2 cup pitted dates
2 tablespoons cocoa powder
1 tablespoon almond butter and Pinch of salt

1. In a food processor, pulse almonds until finely chopped.
2. Add pitted dates, cocoa powder, almond butter, and a pinch of salt.
3. Process until mixture comes together and forms dough.
4. Roll the dough into small balls.
5. Place date balls on a plate and chill in the refrigerator for at least 30 minutes before serving.

Per serving (2 date balls)
Calories: 100|Carbs: 12g| Fats: 6g|Protein: 3g

Blueberry Oatmeal Cookies

Time: 20 min (plus chilling time)| Difficulty: Easy| Serving 2

1/2 cup rolled oats
1/4 cup almond flour and 1/4 cup dried blueberries
2 tbs. honey and 1 tbs. coconut oil, melted
1/2 teaspoon vanilla extract and Pinch of cinnamon

1. Preheat oven to 350°F (175°C) and line a baking sheet with parchment paper.
2. In a bowl, mix together rolled oats, almond flour, dried blueberries, maple syrup or honey, melted coconut oil, vanilla extract, and cinnamon (if using).
3. Form the mixture into small cookies and place them on the prepared baking sheet.
4. Flatten each cookie slightly with the back of a spoon.
5. Bake for 12-15 minutes, or until cookies are golden brown.

Per serving (2 cookies): Calories: 120| Carbs: 15g| Fats: 6g| Protein: 2g

Pumpkin Spice Energy Balls

Time: 20 min (plus chilling time) | Difficulty: Easy | Serving 2

1/2 cup rolled oats and 1/4 cup pumpkin puree
2 tablespoons almond butter
1 tablespoon maple syrup and
Unsweetened shredded coconut for rolling (optional)

1. In a mixing bowl, combine rolled oats, pumpkin puree, almond butter, maple syrup, and pumpkin pie spice.
2. Mix until well combined.
3. Roll the mixture into small balls.
4. Roll each ball in shredded coconut if desired.
5. Place energy balls on a plate and chill in the refrigerator for at least 30 minutes before serving.

Per serving (2 energy balls)
Calories: 100| Carbs: 12g| Fats: 5g| Protein: 2g

Chocolate Covered Strawberries

Time: 15 min (plus chilling time)| Difficulty: Easy| Serving 2

1 cup strawberries, washed and dried
2 ounces dark chocolate, chopped and 1 tsp. coconut oil

1. In a microwave-safe bowl, combine chopped dark chocolate and coconut oil.
2. Microwave in 30-second intervals, stirring between each interval, until chocolate is melted and smooth.
3. Dip each strawberry into the melted chocolate, coating evenly.
4. Place dipped strawberries on a parchment-lined baking sheet.
5. Chill in the refrigerator for at least 30 minutes, or until chocolate is set.

Per serving (5 strawberries)
Calories: 100| Carbs: 12g| Fats: 6g| Protein: 2g

Apple Nachos

Time: 10 minutes| Difficulty: Easy| Serving 2

1 apple, thinly sliced
2 tablespoons almond butter
2 tablespoons dark chocolate chips
Chopped nuts for topping (optional)
Shredded coconut for topping (optional)

1. Arrange apple slices on a serving plate.
2. Drizzle almond butter over the apple slices.
3. Sprinkle dark chocolate chips, chopped nuts, and shredded coconut over the top if desired.

Per serving
Calories: 120| Carbs: 15g| Fats: 7g| Protein: 2g

Peach and Almond Crisp

Time: 45 minutes| Difficulty: Easy| Serving 2

2 ripe peaches, sliced and 1/4 cup almond flour
1/4 cup rolled oats
2 tbs. coconut oil, melted and 2 tbs. honey
1/2 teaspoon cinnamon and Pinch of salt

1. Preheat oven to 350°F (175°C) and grease a baking dish.
2. Place sliced peaches in the prepared baking dish.
3. In a bowl, combine almond flour, rolled oats, melted coconut oil, maple syrup or honey, cinnamon, and a pinch of salt.
4. Sprinkle the mixture over the peaches.
5. Bake for 25-30 minutes, or until topping is golden brown and peaches are bubbly.

Per serving
Calories: 180| Carbs: 20g| Fats: 10g| Protein: 2g

2.9 Pies and Quiches

Chicken Pot Pie

Time: 1 h 15 min| Difficulty: Moderate| Serving 2

1 pre-made pie crust (or homemade)
2 boneless, skinless chicken breasts, cooked and shredded
1 tablespoon olive oil
1 onion, 2 carrots and 2 celery stalks, diced
2 cloves garlic, minced
1/4 cup all-purpose flour
1 cup low-sodium chicken broth and 1 cup frozen peas
1/2 cup milk (or non-dairy milk)

1. Preheat the oven to 375°F (190°C).
2. In a skillet, heat olive oil over medium heat. Add diced onion, carrots, celery, and minced garlic. Cook until softened.
3. Sprinkle flour over the vegetable mixture and stir to coat.
4. Slowly pour in chicken broth and milk, stirring constantly until thickened.
5. Stir in cooked shredded chicken and frozen peas. Season with salt and pepper to taste.
6. Pour the mixture into a pie dish lined with the pre-made pie crust.
7. Cover with another pie crust and crimp the edges to seal. Cut slits in the top crust for ventilation.
8. Bake for 35-40 minutes, or until the crust is golden brown.

Per serving: Calories: 320| Protein: 20g| Fat: 15g| Carbs: 25g

Sweet Potato Shepherd's Pie

Time: 1 hour| Difficulty: Moderate| Serving 2

2 large sweet potatoes, peeled and cubed
1 tablespoon olive oil
1 onion, diced and 2 cloves garlic, minced
1 pound ground turkey
1 cup mixed vegetables (carrots, peas, corn)
1 cup low-sodium chicken broth

1. Preheat the oven to 375°F (190°C) and grease a pie dish.
2. Boil sweet potato cubes in a pot of water until tender. Drain and mash.
3. In a skillet, heat olive oil over medium heat. Add diced onion and minced garlic, cook until softened.
4. Add ground turkey to the skillet and cook until browned.
5. Stir in mixed vegetables and chicken broth. Simmer for 5 minutes.
6. Season with salt and pepper to taste.
7. Transfer the turkey mixture to the greased pie dish.
8. Spread mashed sweet potatoes over the top.
9. Bake for 25-30 minutes, or until the sweet potatoes are golden.

Per serving
Calories: 250| Protein: 20g| Fat: 8g| Carbs: 25g

Cheesy Broccoli Pie

Time: 1 hour| Difficulty: Easy| Serving 2

1 pre-made pie crust (or homemade)
2 cups chopped broccoli florets
1 onion, diced
2 cloves garlic, minced
1 cup shredded cheddar cheese
4 large eggs
1 cup milk (or non-dairy milk)
Salt and pepper to taste

1. Preheat the oven to 375°F (190°C) and grease a pie dish.
2. In a skillet, sauté diced onion and minced garlic until softened.
3. Add chopped broccoli florets to the skillet and cook until tender. Remove from heat and let cool.
4. Sprinkle shredded cheddar cheese over the bottom of the pie crust.
5. In a mixing bowl, whisk together eggs, milk, salt, and pepper.
6. Stir in cooked broccoli mixture.
7. Pour the egg and broccoli mixture into the pie crust.
8. Bake for 35-40 minutes, or until the quiche is set and golden on top.

Per serving
Calories: 250| Protein: 14g| Fat: 15g| Carbs: 18g

Vegetable and Lentil Pie

Time: 1 hour| Difficulty: Moderate| Serving 2

1 pre-made pie crust (or homemade)
1 cup dry green lentils, cooked
1 tablespoon olive oil
1 onion, diced
2 carrots, diced
2 celery stalks, diced
2 cloves garlic, minced
1 cup diced tomatoes
1 cup vegetable broth
1 teaspoon dried thyme

1. Preheat the oven to 375°F (190°C).
2. In a skillet, heat olive oil over medium heat. Add diced onion, carrots, celery, and minced garlic. Cook until softened.
3. Stir in cooked green lentils, diced tomatoes, vegetable broth, dried thyme, salt, and pepper. Simmer for 10-15 minutes.
4. Roll out the pie crust and line a pie dish.
5. Pour the vegetable and lentil mixture into the pie crust.
6. Cover with another pie crust and crimp the edges to seal. Cut slits in the top crust for ventilation.
7. Bake for 30-35 minutes, or until the crust is golden brown.

Per serving
Calories: 290| Protein: 15g| Fat: 12g| Carbs: 30g

Shrimp and Spinach Pie

Time: 1 hour| Difficulty: Moderate| Serving 2

1 pre-made pie crust (or homemade)
1 cup cooked shrimp, chopped
2 cups fresh spinach
1 onion, diced
2 cloves garlic, minced
1 cup shredded mozzarella cheese
4 large eggs
1 cup milk (or non-dairy milk)
Salt and pepper to taste

1. Preheat the oven to 375°F (190°C) and grease a pie dish.
2. In a skillet, sauté diced onion and minced garlic until softened.
3. Add fresh spinach to the skillet and cook until wilted. Remove from heat and let cool.
4. Sprinkle shredded mozzarella cheese over the bottom of the pie crust.
5. Arrange chopped cooked shrimp on top of the cheese.
6. In a mixing bowl, whisk together eggs, milk, salt, and pepper.
7. Stir in cooked spinach mixture.
8. Pour the egg and spinach mixture into the pie crust.
9. Bake for 35-40 minutes, or until the quiche is set and golden on top.

Per serving
Calories: 280| Protein: 16g| Fat: 14g| Carbs: 20g

Chicken and Sweet Potato Pie

Time: 1 h 10 min| Difficulty: Moderate| Serving 2

1 pre-made pie crust
2 cups cooked chicken breast, shredded
1 large sweet potato, peeled and diced
1 onion, chopped
1/2 cup low-sodium chicken broth
1/4 cup skim milk
1 tablespoon olive oil
1 teaspoon dried thyme
Salt and pepper to taste

1. Preheat oven to 375°F (190°C).
2. Sauté onion in olive oil until soft.
3. Add sweet potato, thyme, salt, and pepper. Cook until tender.
4. Stir in chicken, broth, and milk. Cook until thickened.
5. Pour mixture into pie crust.
6. Bake for 35 minutes until crust is golden.

Per serving
Calories: 330| Protein: 18g| Fat: 14g| Carbs: 29g

Turkey and Vegetable Pie

Time: 1 h30 min| Difficulty: Moderate| Serving 2

1 pre-made pie crust (or homemade)
1 tablespoon olive oil
1 onion, diced
2 carrots, diced
2 celery stalks, diced
2 cloves garlic, minced
1 pound ground turkey
1 cup frozen peas
1 cup low-sodium chicken broth
2 tablespoons all-purpose flour

1. Preheat the oven to 375°F (190°C) and grease a pie dish.
2. In a skillet, heat olive oil over medium heat. Add diced onion, carrots, celery, and minced garlic. Cook until softened.
3. Add ground turkey to the skillet and cook until browned.
4. Stir in frozen peas and cook for 2-3 minutes.
5. Sprinkle flour over the turkey mixture and stir to coat.
6. Slowly pour in chicken broth, stirring constantly until thickened.
7. Season with salt and pepper to taste.
8. Transfer the turkey mixture to the greased pie dish.
9. Cover with the pre-made pie crust and crimp the edges to seal. Cut slits in the top crust for ventilation.
10. Bake for 35-40 minutes, or until the crust is golden brown.

Per serving
Calories: 320| Protein: 20g| Fat: 15g| Carbs: 25g

Crab and Corn Pie

Time: 1 hour| Difficulty: Moderate| Serving 2

1 pre-made pie crust (or homemade)
1 cup lump crab meat
1 cup corn kernels
1 onion, diced
2 cloves garlic, minced
1 cup shredded cheddar cheese
4 large eggs
1 cup milk (or non-dairy milk)
Salt and pepper to taste

1. Preheat the oven to 375°F (190°C) and grease a pie dish.
2. In a skillet, sauté diced onion and minced garlic until softened.
3. Add corn kernels to the skillet and cook until slightly caramelized.
4. Stir in lump crab meat and cook until heated through. Remove from heat and let cool.
5. Sprinkle shredded cheddar cheese over the bottom of the pie crust.
6. Arrange the crab and corn mixture on top of the cheese.
7. In a mixing bowl, whisk together eggs, milk, salt, and pepper.
8. Pour the egg mixture over the crab and corn mixture in the pie dish.
9. Bake for 35-40 minutes, or until the quiche is set and golden on top.

Per serving
Calories: 310| Protein: 16g| Fat: 16g| Carbs: 22g

Cod and Vegetable Pie

Time: 1 hour| Difficulty: Moderate| Serving 2

1 pre-made pie crust (or homemade)
2 cod fillets, cooked and flaked
1 cup diced potatoes
1 onion, diced
2 carrots, diced
1 cup frozen peas
1 cup low-sodium chicken broth
2 tablespoons all-purpose flour
1/2 cup heavy cream

1. Preheat the oven to 375°F (190°C) and grease a pie dish.
2. In a skillet, sauté diced onion until softened.
3. Add diced potatoes and carrots to the skillet and cook until slightly tender.
4. Stir in cooked and flaked cod fillets and frozen peas.
5. Sprinkle flour over the cod and vegetable mixture and stir to coat.
6. Slowly pour in chicken broth and heavy cream, stirring constantly until thickened.
7. Season with salt and pepper to taste.
8. Transfer the cod and vegetable mixture to the greased pie dish.
9. Cover with the pre-made pie crust and crimp the edges to seal. Cut slits in the top crust for ventilation.
10. Bake for 35-40 minutes, or until the crust is golden brown.

Per serving
Calories: 340| Protein: 18g| Fat: 18g| Carbs: 25g

Tuna and Olive Pie

Time: 50 minutes| Difficulty: Easy| Serving 2

1 pre-made pie crust
1 can tuna, drained
1/2 cup black olives, sliced
1/4 cup low-fat cream cheese
1/4 cup low-fat milk
2 eggs
Salt and pepper to taste

1. Preheat oven to 375°F (190°C).
2. In a bowl, mix tuna, olives, cream cheese, milk, eggs, salt, and pepper.
3. Pour into pie crust.
4. Bake for 30-35 minutes until set.

Per serving
Calories: 280| Protein: 18g| Fat: 16g| Carbs: 18g

Salmon and Broccoli Pie

Time: 1 hour| Difficulty: Moderate| Serving 2

1 pre-made pie crust (or homemade)
2 salmon fillets, cooked and flaked
2 cups chopped broccoli florets
1 onion, diced and 2 cloves garlic, minced
1 cup shredded cheddar cheese
4 large eggs and 1 cup milk (or non-dairy milk)

1. Preheat the oven to 375°F (190°C) and grease a pie dish.
2. In a skillet, sauté diced onion and minced garlic until softened.
3. Add chopped broccoli florets to the skillet and cook until tender. Remove from heat and let cool.
4. Sprinkle shredded cheddar cheese over the bottom of the pie crust.
5. Arrange cooked and flaked salmon on top of the cheese.
6. In a mixing bowl, whisk together eggs, milk, salt, and pepper.
7. Stir in cooked broccoli mixture.
8. Pour the egg and broccoli mixture into the pie crust.
9. Bake for 35-40 minutes, or until the quiche is set and golden on top.

Per serving
Calories: 300| Protein: 18g| Fat: 16g| Carbs: 20g

Tuna and Mushroom Pie

Time: 1 hour| Difficulty: Moderate| Serving 2

1 pre-made pie crust (or homemade)
1 can tuna, drained and flaked
2 cups sliced mushrooms
1 onion, diced
2 cloves garlic, minced
1 cup shredded Swiss cheese
4 large eggs
1 cup milk (or non-dairy milk)
Salt and pepper to taste

1. Preheat the oven to 375°F (190°C) and grease a pie dish.
2. In a skillet, sauté diced onion and minced garlic until softened.
3. Add sliced mushrooms to the skillet and cook until tender. Remove from heat and let cool.
4. Sprinkle shredded Swiss cheese over the bottom of the pie crust.
5. Arrange flaked tuna and cooked mushroom mixture on top of the cheese.
6. In a mixing bowl, whisk together eggs, milk, salt, and pepper.
7. Pour the egg mixture over the tuna and mushroom mixture in the pie dish.
8. Bake for 35-40 minutes, or until the quiche is set and golden on top.

Per serving
Calories: 290| Protein: 16g| Fat: 15g| Carbs: 20g

Shrimp and Asparagus Quiche

Time: 1 hour| Difficulty: Moderate| Serving 2

1 pre-made pie crust
1 cup asparagus, chopped
1 cup shrimp, cooked and chopped
1/2 cup low-fat cream cheese
1/4 cup low-fat milk
4 eggs
1 tablespoon olive oil
Salt and pepper to taste

1. Preheat oven to 375°F (190°C).
2. Sauté asparagus in olive oil until tender.
3. In a bowl, whisk together eggs, milk, cream cheese, salt, and pepper.
4. Stir in asparagus and shrimp.
5. Pour into pie crust.
6. Bake for 35-40 minutes until set.

Per serving: Calories: 280| Protein: 16g| Fat: 16g| Carbs: 18g

Sweet Corn and Chicken Pie

Time: 1 hour| Difficulty: Moderate| Serving 2

1 pre-made pie crust
2 cups cooked chicken, shredded
1 cup sweet corn
1/2 cup low-fat cheddar cheese, shredded
1/4 cup skim milk
4 eggs
1 tablespoon olive oil

1. Preheat oven to 375°F (190°C).
2. In a bowl, whisk together eggs, milk, salt, and pepper.
3. Stir in chicken, corn, and cheese.
4. Pour into pie crust.
5. Bake for 35-40 minutes until set.

Per serving: Calories: 300| Protein: 18g| Fat: 16g| Carbs: 20g

Broccoli and Cheddar Quiche

Time: 1 hour| Difficulty: Easy| Serving 2

1 pre-made pie crust
2 cups broccoli, chopped and blanched
1/2 cup low-fat cheddar cheese, shredded
1/4 cup skim milk
4 eggs

1. Preheat oven to 375°F (190°C).
2. Spread broccoli and cheese in pie crust.
3. In a bowl, whisk together eggs, milk, salt, and pepper.
4. Pour over broccoli.
5. Bake for 35-40 minutes until set.

Per serving: Calories: 250| Protein: 12g| Fat: 14g| Carbs: 18g

Beef and Mushroom Pie

Time: 1 h20 min| Difficulty: Moderate| Serving 2

1 pre-made pie crust
2 cups lean ground beef, cooked
1 cup mushrooms, sliced
1 onion, chopped
1/2 cup low-sodium beef broth
1/4 cup skim milk
2 tablespoons all-purpose flour
1 tablespoon Worcestershire sauce
1 tablespoon olive oil
Salt and pepper to taste

1. Preheat oven to 375°F (190°C).
2. Sauté onion and mushrooms in olive oil until soft.
3. Add cooked beef, Worcestershire sauce, and flour. Stir until well combined.
4. Slowly add broth and milk, stirring until thickened.
5. Pour into pie crust.
6. Bake for 35-40 minutes until crust is golden.

Per serving
Calories: 320| Protein: 20g| Fat: 17g| Carbs: 20g

Peach and Berry Cobbler

Time: 50 minutes| Difficulty: Easy| Serving 2

2 cups fresh peaches, sliced
1 cup mixed berries (blueberries, raspberries)
1/2 cup whole wheat flour
1/2 cup rolled oats
1/4 cup brown sugar
1/4 cup unsalted butter, melted
1/2 teaspoon cinnamon
1/4 teaspoon nutmeg

1. Preheat oven to 375°F (190°C).
2. Arrange fruit in a baking dish.
3. In a bowl, mix flour, oats, sugar, cinnamon, nutmeg, and butter until crumbly.
4. Sprinkle over fruit.
5. Bake for 30-35 minutes until topping is golden.

Per serving
Calories: 210| Protein: 3g| Fat: 8g| Carbs: 34g

Lemon and Herb Salmon Pie

Time: 50 minutes| Difficulty: Moderate| Serving 2

1 pre-made pie crust
2 salmon fillets, cooked and flaked
1/4 cup low-fat cream cheese
1 lemon, zest and juice
1 tablespoon dill, chopped
1 tablespoon parsley, chopped
2 green onions, chopped
Salt and pepper to taste

1. Preheat oven to 375°F (190°C).
2. In a bowl, mix flaked salmon, cream cheese, lemon zest, lemon juice, dill, parsley, green onions, salt, and pepper.
3. Spread salmon mixture into pie crust.
4. Bake for 30-35 minutes until crust is golden.

Per serving
Calories: 290| Protein: 18g| Fat: 15g| Carbs: 20g

Lobster Pot Pie

Time: 1 h 30 min| Difficulty: Moderate| Serving 2

1 pre-made pie crust (or homemade)
1 cup cooked lobster meat, chopped
2 cups diced potatoes
1 onion, diced
2 cloves garlic, minced
1 cup frozen peas
1 cup low-sodium chicken broth
2 tablespoons all-purpose flour
1/2 cup heavy cream
Salt and pepper to taste

1. Preheat the oven to 375°F (190°C) and grease a pie dish.
2. In a skillet, sauté diced onion and minced garlic until softened.
3. Add diced potatoes to the skillet and cook until slightly tender.
4. Stir in chopped cooked lobster meat and frozen peas.
5. Sprinkle flour over the lobster mixture and stir to coat.
6. Slowly pour in chicken broth and heavy cream, stirring constantly until thickened.
7. Season with salt and pepper to taste.
8. Transfer the lobster mixture to the greased pie dish.
9. Cover with the pre-made pie crust and crimp the edges to seal. Cut slits in the top crust for ventilation.
10. Bake for 35-40 minutes, or until the crust is golden brown.

Per serving
Calories: 350| Protein: 18g| Fat: 20g| Carbs: 25g

Turkey and Sweet Potato Shepherd's Pie

Time: 50 minutes| Difficulty: Easy| Serving 2

2 cups cooked, ground turkey breast
2 sweet potatoes, mashed
1 cup frozen mixed vegetables (carrots, peas, corn)
1 onion, chopped
1 clove garlic, minced and 1 tbsp. olive oil
1/2 cup low-sodium chicken broth

1. Preheat oven to 375°F (190°C).
2. Sauté onion and garlic in olive oil until translucent.
3. Add ground turkey and vegetables. Cook for 5 minutes.
4. Add broth and simmer until mostly absorbed.
5. Place turkey mixture in a baking dish, top with mashed sweet potatoes.
6. Bake for 20 minutes until topping is slightly crispy.

Per serving: Calories: 280| Protein: 21g| Fat: 10g| Carbs: 25g

Chicken and Leek Pie

Time: 1 hour| Difficulty: Moderate| Serving 2

1 pre-made pie crust
2 cups cooked chicken breast, shredded
2 leeks, cleaned and sliced
1/2 cup low-fat cream cheese
1/4 cup low-fat milk
1 tbsp. olive oil

1. Preheat oven to 375°F (190°C).
2. Sauté leeks in olive oil until soft.
3. Mix leeks, chicken, cream cheese, milk, salt, and pepper.
4. Pour mixture into pie crust.
5. Bake for 30-35 minutes until crust is golden.

Per serving: Calories: 290\ Protein: 19g| Fat: 16g| Carbs: 18g

Salmon and Asparagus Quiche

Time: 1 hour| Difficulty: Moderate| Serving 2

1 pre-made pie crust
1 cup cooked salmon, flaked
1 cup asparagus, chopped
1/2 cup low-fat cream cheese
1/4 cup skim milk
4 eggs

1. Preheat oven to 375°F (190°C).
2. Spread salmon and asparagus in pie crust.
3. In a bowl, whisk together eggs, cream cheese, milk, salt, and pepper.
4. Pour over salmon and asparagus.
5. Bake for 35-40 minutes until set.

Per serving
Calories: 280| Protein: 20g| Fat: 16g| Carbs: 12g

Beef and Potato Pie

Time: 1 h20 min| Difficulty: Moderate| Serving 2

1 pre-made pie crust
2 cups lean ground beef
2 potatoes, boiled and mashed
1 carrot and 1 onion, finely chopped
1/2 cup peas
1/2 cup low-sodium beef broth
1 tbsp. olive oil

1. Preheat oven to 375°F (190°C).
2. Cook beef and onion in olive oil until browned.
3. Add carrots, peas, and broth, simmer until veggies are tender.
4. Place beef mixture in pie crust, top with mashed potatoes.
5. Bake for 40 minutes until topping is golden.

Per serving
Calories: 300| Protein: 20g| Fat: 15g| Carbs: 20g

Chicken and Broccoli Pie

Time: 1 hour| Difficulty: Moderate| Serving 2

1 pre-made pie crust
2 cups cooked chicken breast, chopped
1 cup broccoli florets
1/2 cup low-fat cream cheese
1/4 cup skim milk
Salt and pepper to taste

1. Preheat oven to 375°F (190°C).
2. Blanch broccoli until just tender.
3. Mix chicken, broccoli, cream cheese, and milk. Season with salt and pepper.
4. Pour into pie crust.
5. Bake for 35-40 minutes until golden and set.

Per serving
Calories: 280| Protein: 25g| Fat: 14g| Carbs: 12g

2.10 Smoothies and Beverages Recipes

Green Smoothie Bowl

Time: 5 minutes| Difficulty: Easy| Serving 2

2 cups baby spinach
1 ripe banana
1 cup frozen mixed berries
1/2 cup almond milk
2 tablespoons chia seeds
Toppings: sliced fruit, nuts, seeds, granola (optional)
1. In a blender, combine baby spinach, banana, frozen mixed berries, almond milk, and chia seeds.
2. Blend until smooth and creamy.
3. Divide the smoothie mixture between two serving bowls.
4. Top with sliced fruit, nuts, seeds, or granola, if desired.
5. Enjoy this nutrient-packed and refreshing breakfast bowl!

Per serving: Calories: 200| Protein: 5g| Carbs: 30g| Fat: 8g| Fiber: 8g

---

Strawberry Banana Smoothie

Time: 5 minutes| Difficulty: Easy| Serving 2

1 cup strawberries, hulled
1 banana
1 cup Greek yogurt
1/2 cup almond milk
Honey, to taste (optional)
1. Place all the ingredients in a blender.
2. Blend until smooth and creamy.
3. Taste and adjust sweetness with honey if desired.
4. Pour into glasses and serve immediately.

Per serving
Calories: 150| Protein: 10g| Carbs: 20g| Fat: 3g| Fiber: 4g

Banana Almond Milkshake

Time: 5 minutes| Difficulty: Easy| Serving 2

2 ripe bananas
1 cup unsweetened almond milk
2 tablespoons almond butter
1 tablespoon honey or maple syrup
1/2 teaspoon vanilla extract and Ice cubes
1. Combine bananas, almond milk, almond butter, honey or maple syrup, vanilla extract, and ice cubes in a blender.
2. Blend until smooth and creamy.
3. Pour into glasses and serve immediately.

Per serving: Calories: 180| Carbs: 25g| Fats: 7g| Protein: 5g

Turmeric Ginger Smoothie

Time: 5 minutes| Difficulty: Easy| Serving 2

1 ripe banana
1 cup frozen mango chunks
1 cup spinach leaves
1/2 cup Greek yogurt
1 teaspoon grated fresh ginger
1/2 teaspoon ground turmeric
1 cup almond milk
Honey or maple syrup for sweetening (optional)

1. In a blender, combine banana, frozen mango chunks, spinach leaves, Greek yoghurt, grated fresh ginger, ground turmeric, and almond milk.
2. Blend until smooth and creamy.
3. Sweeten with honey or maple syrup, if desired.
4. Pour into glasses and serve immediately.
5. Enjoy this vibrant and immune-boosting smoothie!

Per serving: Calories: 250| Protein: 10g| Carbs: 40g| Fat: 5g| Fiber: 6g

Matcha Green Tea Latte

Time: 5 minutes| Difficulty: Easy| Serving 2

2 teaspoons matcha green tea powder
1 cup hot water
1 cup unsweetened almond milk
Honey or stevia (optional, to taste)

1. Whisk matcha powder into hot water until dissolved.
2. Heat almond milk in a saucepan until hot but not boiling.
3. Froth almond milk using a frother or whisk.
4. Pour matcha mixture into mugs.
5. Top with frothed almond milk.
6. Sweeten with honey or stevia if desired.

Per serving: Calories: 15| Carbs: 2g| Fats: 1g| Protein: 1g

Berry Blast Smoothie

Time: 5 minutes| Difficulty: Easy| Serving 2

1 cup mixed berries (such as strawberries, blueberries, raspberries)
1/2 cup plain Greek yogurt
1 ripe banana
1 tablespoon chia seeds
1 cup almond milk
Handful of ice cubes

1. Place all ingredients in a blender.
2. Blend until smooth and well combined.
3. Pour into glasses and serve immediately.

Per serving
Calories: 150| Carbs: 20g| Fats: 5g| Protein: 7g

Creamy Almond Butter Smoothie

Time: 5 minutes| Difficulty: Easy| Serving 2

2 tablespoons almond butter
1 ripe banana
1 cup unsweetened almond milk
1 tablespoon honey or maple syrup
1/2 teaspoon vanilla extract
Handful of spinach (optional)
Handful of ice cubes

1. Combine all ingredients in a blender.
2. Blend until smooth and creamy.
3. Pour into glasses and serve immediately.

Per serving
Calories: 200| Carbs: 25g| Fats: 10g| Protein: 5g

Tropical Paradise Smoothie

Time: 5 minutes| Difficulty: Easy| Serving 2

1/2 cup frozen pineapple chunks
1/2 cup frozen mango chunks and 1/2 banana
1/2 cup coconut milk and 1/2 cup orange juice
Handful of spinach (optional)
Handful of ice cubes

1. Add all ingredients to a blender.
2. Blend until smooth and creamy.
3. Pour into glasses and enjoy immediately.

Per serving: Calories: 160| Carbs: 30g| Fats: 5g| Protein: 2g

Peaches and Cream Smoothie

Time: 5 minutes| Difficulty: Easy| Serving 2

1 cup frozen peach slices
1/2 cup plain Greek yogurt
1/2 cup unsweetened almond milk
1 tablespoon honey or maple syrup
1/2 teaspoon vanilla extract
Handful of ice cubes

1. Place all ingredients in a blender.
2. Blend until smooth and creamy.
3. Pour into glasses and serve immediately.

Per serving
Calories: 150| Carbs: 20g| Fats: 3g| Protein: 8g

Pineapple Coconut Smoothie

Time: 5 minutes| Difficulty: Easy| Serving 2

1 cup frozen pineapple chunks
1/2 cup coconut milk
1/2 cup plain Greek yogurt
Honey or stevia (optional, to taste)and Ice cubes

1.   Place all ingredients in a blender.
2.   Blend until smooth and creamy.
3.   Sweeten with honey or stevia if desired.
4.   Pour into glasses and serve immediately.

Per serving
Calories: 150| Carbs: 20g|Fats: 3g| Protein: 8g

Green Goddess Smoothie

Time: 5 minutes| Difficulty: Easy| Serving 2

2 cups spinach and 1 ripe banana
1/2 cup cucumber, chopped
1/2 avocado
1 cup coconut water and Juice of 1/2 lime
Handful of ice cubes

1.   Combine all ingredients in a blender.
2.   Blend until smooth and creamy.
3.   Pour into glasses and serve immediately.

Per serving
Calories: 120|Carbs: 20g| Fats: 5g| Protein: 3

Banana Nut Smoothie

Time: 5 minutes| Difficulty: Easy| Serving 2

2 ripe bananas
2 tablespoons almond butter
1 cup unsweetened almond milk
1 tablespoon honey or maple syrup
1/2 teaspoon cinnamon
Handful of ice cubes

1.   Add all ingredients to a blender.
2.   Blend until smooth and creamy.
3.   Pour into glasses and enjoy immediately.

Per serving
Calories: 220| Carbs: 30g| Fats: 10g| Protein: 5g

Peanut Butter Banana Smoothie

Time: 5 minutes| Difficulty: Easy| Serving 2

2 ripe bananas
2 tablespoons peanut butter
1 cup unsweetened almond milk
1 tablespoon honey or maple syrup
Handful of ice cubes

1. Place all ingredients in a blender.
2. Blend until smooth and creamy.
3. Pour into glasses and enjoy immediately.

Per serving
Calories: 220| Carbs: 25g| Fats: 10g| Protein: 5g

Peach Green Tea Smoothie

Time: 5 minutes| Difficulty: Easy| Serving 2

1 cup frozen peach slices
1 cup brewed green tea, chilled
1/2 cup plain Greek yogurt
Honey or stevia (optional, to taste)
Ice cubes

1. Combine peach slices, green tea, Greek yogurt, and honey or stevia in a blender.
2. Blend until smooth and creamy.
3. Add ice cubes and blend until desired consistency.
4. Pour into glasses and serve immediately.

Per serving
Calories: 120| Carbs: 20g| Fats: 1g| Protein: 8g

Mango Coconut Smoothie

Time: 5 minutes| Difficulty: Easy| Serving 2

1 cup frozen mango chunks
1/2 cup coconut milk
1/2 cup plain Greek yogurt
1 tablespoon honey or maple syrup
Juice of 1/2 lime
Handful of ice cubes

1. Add all ingredients to a blender.
2. Blend until smooth and creamy.
3. Pour into glasses and serve immediately.

Per serving
Calories: 160| Carbs: 20g| Fats: 7g| Protein: 7g

Vanilla Berry Smoothie

Time: 5 minutes| Difficulty: Easy| Serving 2

1 cup mixed berries (such as strawberries, raspberries, blueberries)
1/2 cup plain Greek yogurt
1/2 cup unsweetened almond milk
1 tablespoon honey or maple syrup
1/2 teaspoon vanilla extract
Handful of ice cubes

1. Combine all ingredients in a blender.
2. Blend until smooth and creamy.
3. Pour into glasses and serve immediately.

Per serving
Calories: 150| Carbs: 20g| Fats: 3g| Protein: 8g

Mixed Berry Smoothie Bowl

Time: 10 minutes| Difficulty: Easy| Serving 2

1 cup mixed berries (such as strawberries, blueberries, raspberries)
1/2 banana
1/2 cup plain Greek yogurt
1/4 cup almond milk
1 tablespoon chia seeds
Toppings: *sliced fruit, granola, shredded coconut*

1. Place mixed berries, banana, Greek yogurt, almond milk, and chia seeds in a blender.
2. Blend until smooth and creamy.
3. Pour into bowls.
4. Top with sliced fruit, granola, and shredded coconut.
5. Serve immediately.

Per serving
Calories: 150|Carbs: 20g| Fats: 3g| Protein: 8g

Chapter 3: Special Occasion Recipes

3.1 Festive and Holiday Dishes

Garlic Butter Roasted Rack of Lamb

Time: 1 hour| Difficulty: Moderate| Serving 2

1 rack of lamb (about 1 lb.)
4 cloves garlic, minced
2 tablespoons fresh rosemary, chopped
2 tablespoons unsalted butter, melted
Salt and pepper to taste

1. Preheat the oven to 400°F (200°C).
2. In a small bowl, mix together minced garlic, chopped rosemary, melted butter, salt, and pepper.
3. Rub the garlic butter mixture all over the rack of lamb.
4. Place the rack of lamb in a roasting pan.
5. Roast in the preheated oven for about 25-30 minutes, or until the lamb is cooked to your desired doneness (medium-rare is recommended), with an internal temperature of 145°F (63°C).
6. Let the lamb rest for 10 minutes before slicing.
7. Serve hot as a festive main dish.

Per serving
Calories: 350| Carbs: 0g| Fats: 25g| Protein: 30g

Maple Mustard Glazed Salmon

Time: 30 minutes| Difficulty: Easy| Serving 2

2 salmon fillets
1/4 cup maple syrup
2 tablespoons Dijon mustard
1 tablespoon olive oil
Salt and pepper to taste

1. Preheat the oven to 400°F (200°C).
2. In a small bowl, mix together maple syrup, Dijon mustard, olive oil, salt, and pepper.
3. Place the salmon fillets on a baking sheet lined with parchment paper.
4. Brush the maple mustard glaze all over the salmon fillets.
5. Roast in the preheated oven for about 12-15 minutes, or until the salmon is cooked through and flakes easily with a fork.
6. Serve hot as a festive main dish.

Per serving
Calories: 300| Carbs: 20g| Fats: 15g| Protein: 30g

Roasted Turkey Breast with Herbs

Time: 1 hour| Difficulty: Moderate| Serving 2

1 turkey breast (about 1.5 lbs.)
2 tablespoons olive oil
2 cloves garlic, minced
1 teaspoon dried thyme
1 teaspoon dried rosemary
Salt and pepper to taste

1. Preheat the oven to 375°F (190°C).
2. In a small bowl, mix together the olive oil, minced garlic, dried thyme, dried rosemary, salt, and pepper.
3. Rub the mixture all over the turkey breast.
4. Place the turkey breast on a baking sheet lined with parchment paper.
5. Roast in the preheated oven for about 45-50 minutes, or until the internal temperature reaches 165°F (74°C).
6. Remove from the oven and let it rest for 10 minutes before slicing.
7. Serve with your favorite side dishes.

Per serving
Calories: 250| Carbs: 1g| Fats: 11g| Protein: 35g

Rosemary Garlic Roast Chicken

Time: 1 h 30 min| Difficulty: Moderate| Serving 2

1 whole chicken (about 3-4 lbs.)
4 cloves garlic, minced
2 tablespoons fresh rosemary, chopped
2 tablespoons olive oil
Salt and pepper to taste

1. Preheat the oven to 375°F (190°C).
2. In a small bowl, mix together minced garlic, chopped rosemary, olive oil, salt, and pepper to form a paste.
3. Rub the garlic-rosemary paste all over the chicken, including under the skin.
4. Place the chicken in a roasting pan or on a baking sheet.
5. Roast in the preheated oven for about 1 hour and 15 minutes, or until the chicken is golden brown and the internal temperature reaches 165°F (75°C).
6. Let the chicken rest for 10 minutes before carving.
7. Serve hot as a festive main dish.

Per serving
Calories: 300| Carbs: 0g| Fats: 15g| Protein: 40g

Garlic Herb Roasted Pork Tenderloin

Time: 1 hour| Difficulty: Moderate| Serving 2

1 pork tenderloin (about 1 lb.)
4 cloves garlic, minced
2 tablespoons fresh herbs (such as rosemary, thyme, or sage), chopped
2 tablespoons olive oil
Salt and pepper to taste

1. Preheat the oven to 400°F (200°C).
2. In a small bowl, mix together minced garlic, chopped fresh herbs, olive oil, salt, and pepper.
3. Rub the garlic-herb mixture all over the pork tenderloin.
4. Place the pork tenderloin in a roasting pan or on a baking sheet.
5. Roast in the preheated oven for about 25-30 minutes, or until the pork is cooked through and the internal temperature reaches 145°F (63°C).
6. Let the pork tenderloin rest for 10 minutes before slicing.
7. Serve hot as a festive main dish.

Per serving
Calories: 280| Carbs: 1g| Fats: 10g| Protein: 45g

Cranberry Glazed Turkey Breast

Time: 2 hours| Difficulty: Moderate| Serving 2

1 turkey breast (about 2 lbs.)
1/2 cup cranberry juice
1/4 cup honey
2 tablespoons balsamic vinegar
1 tablespoon olive oil
Salt and pepper to taste

1. Preheat the oven to 375°F (190°C).
2. In a small saucepan, combine cranberry juice, honey, balsamic vinegar, olive oil, salt, and pepper. Bring to a boil, then reduce heat and simmer until slightly thickened, about 10-15 minutes.
3. Place the turkey breast in a roasting pan or on a baking sheet.
4. Brush the cranberry glaze all over the turkey breast.
5. Roast in the preheated oven for about 1 hour and 30 minutes, or until the turkey is cooked through and the internal temperature reaches 165°F (75°C), basting with the glaze every 30 minutes.
6. Let the turkey breast rest for 10 minutes before slicing.
7. Serve hot as a festive main dish.

Per serving
Calories: 250| Carbs: 20g|Fats: 5g| Protein: 35g

Beef Stew with Root Vegetables

Time: 2 hours| Difficulty: Medium| Serving 2

1 lb. lean beef stew meat, cut into cubes
1 tbsp. olive oil
2 carrots, diced
2 parsnips, diced
1 turnip, diced
4 cups beef broth (low-fat)
1 onion, chopped
2 cloves garlic, minced
1 tsp. dried thyme
Salt and pepper, to taste

1. Heat olive oil in a large pot and brown the beef on all sides.
2. Add onions and garlic, cook until softened.
3. Add carrots, parsnips, turnip, thyme, and beef broth.
4. Bring to a boil, then reduce to a simmer.
5. Cover and simmer for 1.5 hours or until meat is tender.

Per serving
Calories: 280| Protein: 25g| Fat: 10g| Carbs: 22g

Balsamic Glazed Ham

Time: 2 hours| Difficulty: Moderate| Serving 2

1 small boneless ham (about 2 lbs.)
1/4 cup balsamic vinegar
2 tablespoons honey
1 tablespoon Dijon mustard
1 tablespoon olive oil
Salt and pepper to taste

1. Preheat the oven to 350°F (175°C).
2. In a small saucepan, combine balsamic vinegar, honey, Dijon mustard, olive oil, salt, and pepper. Bring to a boil, then reduce heat and simmer until slightly thickened, about 10-15 minutes.
3. Place the ham in a roasting pan.
4. Brush the balsamic glaze all over the ham.
5. Roast in the preheated oven for about 1 hour, or until the ham is heated through.
6. Baste the ham with the glaze every 20 minutes.
7. Serve hot as a festive main dish.

Per serving
Calories: 300| Carbs: 10g| Fats: 10g| Protein: 45g

Apple Cider Glazed Pork Chops

Time: 1 hour| Difficulty: Moderate| Serving 2

2 pork chops
1/2 cup apple cider
2 tablespoons apple cider vinegar
2 tablespoons honey
1 tablespoon Dijon mustard
1 tablespoon olive oil
Salt and pepper to taste

1. In a small saucepan, combine apple cider, apple cider vinegar, honey, Dijon mustard, olive oil, salt, and pepper. Bring to a boil, then reduce heat and simmer until slightly thickened, about 10-15 minutes.
2. Preheat a skillet over medium-high heat and add a little olive oil.
3. Season the pork chops with salt and pepper on both sides.
4. Sear the pork chops in the skillet for about 3-4 minutes on each side, until golden brown.
5. Reduce heat to medium-low and pour the apple cider glaze over the pork chops.
6. Continue to cook for another 5-7 minutes, or until the pork chops are cooked through and the glaze is caramelized.

Per serving
Calories: 280| Carbs: 20g| Fats: 10g| Protein: 30g

Cider Glazed Pork Roast

Time: 2 hours| Difficulty: Moderate| Serving 2

1 pork shoulder roast (about 2 lbs.)
1 cup apple cider
1/4 cup apple cider vinegar
2 tablespoons brown sugar
1 tablespoon Dijon mustard
1 tablespoon olive oil

1. Preheat the oven to 325°F (160°C).
2. In a small saucepan, combine apple cider, apple cider vinegar, brown sugar, Dijon mustard, olive oil, salt, and pepper. Heat over medium heat until well combined.
3. Place the pork shoulder roast in a roasting pan.
4. Pour the cider glaze over the pork shoulder roast.
5. Roast in the preheated oven for about 2 hours, or until the pork is tender and pulls apart easily.
6. Baste the pork shoulder roast with the glaze every 30 minutes.

Per serving
Calories: 300| Carbs: 25g| Fats: 15g| Protein: 35g

Herb Crusted Beef Tenderloin

Time: 1 h 30 min| Difficulty: Moderate| Serving 2

1 beef tenderloin (about 1 lb.)
2 tablespoons fresh thyme leaves
2 tablespoons fresh rosemary, chopped
2 tablespoons fresh parsley, chopped
2 tablespoons Dijon mustard
2 tablespoons olive oil
Salt and pepper to taste

1. Preheat the oven to 425°F (220°C).
2. In a small bowl, mix together fresh thyme leaves, chopped rosemary, chopped parsley, Dijon mustard, olive oil, salt, and pepper.
3. Rub the herb mixture all over the beef tenderloin.
4. Place the beef tenderloin on a baking sheet.
5. Roast in the preheated oven for about 25-30 minutes, or until the beef tenderloin reaches your desired level of doneness (medium-rare is recommended), with an internal temperature of 145°F (63°C).
6. Let the beef tenderloin rest for 10 minutes before slicing.

Per serving
Calories: 350| Carbs: 0g| Fats: 20g| Protein: 40g

Cranberry Pecan Stuffed Pork Chops

Time: 1 h 30 min| Difficulty: Moderate| Serving 2

2 pork chops
1/4 cup dried cranberries, chopped
1/4 cup pecans, chopped
2 tablespoons breadcrumbs
2 tablespoons olive oil
Salt and pepper to taste

1. Preheat the oven to 375°F (190°C).
2. In a small bowl, mix together chopped dried cranberries, chopped pecans, breadcrumbs, olive oil, salt, and pepper.
3. Using a sharp knife, cut a slit horizontally in each pork chop to create a pocket.
4. Stuff each pork chop with the cranberry pecan mixture, pressing gently to seal.
5. Heat a skillet over medium-high heat and add a little olive oil.
6. Sear the stuffed pork chops for about 3-4 minutes on each side, until golden brown.
7. Transfer the seared pork chops to a baking dish and bake in the preheated oven for about 20-25 minutes, or until cooked through.
8. Serve hot as a festive main dish.

Per serving
Calories: 350| Carbs: 15g| Fats: 20g| Protein: 30g

Apricot Glazed Pork Loin

Time: 1 h30 min| Difficulty: Moderate| Serving 2

1 pork loin roasts (about 2 lbs.)
1/2 cup apricot preserves
2 tablespoons soy sauce
2 tablespoons olive oil
2 cloves garlic, minced
Salt and pepper to taste

1. Preheat the oven to 375°F (190°C).
2. In a small saucepan, combine apricot preserves, soy sauce, olive oil, minced garlic, salt, and pepper. Heat over medium heat until melted and well combined.
3. Place the pork loin roast in a roasting pan.
4. Brush the apricot glaze all over the pork loin.
5. Roast in the preheated oven for about 1 hour and 15 minutes, or until the pork loin is cooked through and the internal temperature reaches 145°F (63°C), basting with the glaze every 20 minutes.
6. Let the pork loin rest for 10 minutes before slicing.
7. Serve hot as a festive main dish.

Per serving
Calories: 320| Carbs: 20g| Fats: 15g| Protein: 35g

Baked Chicken with Spinach and Pine Nuts

Time: 40 minutes| Difficulty: Easy| Serving 2

2 chicken breasts (6 oz. each)
2 cups fresh spinach
2 tablespoons pine nuts
1 lemon, juiced and zested
2 cloves garlic, minced
Salt and pepper to taste
1 tablespoon olive oil

1. Preheat the oven to 400°F.
2. In a pan, sauté spinach with garlic until wilted.
3. Mix in pine nuts, lemon zest, and juice.
4. Slice chicken breasts halfway to create a pocket, stuff with spinach mixture.
5. Place on a baking sheet, drizzle with olive oil, and season with salt and pepper.
6. Bake for 25-30 minutes until chicken is cooked through.

Per serving
Calories: 310| Protein: 35g| Fat: 14g| Carbs: 8g

Herb-Crusted Rack of Lamb

Time: 45 minutes| Difficulty: Medium| Serving 2

1 rack of lamb (about 1 lb., trimmed of fat)
1 tablespoon Dijon mustard
1/4 cup breadcrumbs
1 tablespoon chopped fresh rosemary
1 tablespoon chopped fresh thyme
2 cloves garlic, minced
Salt and pepper to taste
1 tablespoon olive oil

1. Preheat the oven to 400°F.
2. Season the lamb with salt and pepper.
3. Rub Dijon mustard all over the lamb.
4. Mix breadcrumbs, rosemary, thyme, and garlic, then press onto the lamb.
5. Heat olive oil in an ovenproof skillet, sear lamb on all sides.
6. Transfer skillet to the oven and roast for 20-25 minutes for medium-rare.
7. Let rest before carving.

Per serving
Calories: 320| Protein: 22g| Fat: 24g| Carbs: 4g

Veal Scallopini with Mushroom Sauce

Time: 30 minutes| Difficulty: Medium| Serving 2

4 veal cutlets (4 oz. each)
1 cup sliced mushrooms
1/2 cup low-sodium chicken broth
1/4 cup white wine (optional)
1 tablespoon capers
1 tablespoon lemon juice
1 tablespoon chopped parsley
1 tablespoon olive oil
Salt and pepper to taste

1. Heat olive oil in a large skillet over medium heat.
2. Season veal cutlets with salt and pepper, sear for 1-2 minutes on each side.
3. Remove veal and set aside.
4. Add mushrooms to the skillet, sauté until golden.
5. Deglaze with chicken broth and white wine, simmer for 5 minutes.
6. Stir in capers and lemon juice.
7. Return veal to the skillet; simmer for another 2-3 minutes.
8. Garnish with parsley before serving.

Per serving
Calories: 220| Protein: 24g| Fat: 9g| Carbs: 5g

Pork Tenderloin with Apples and Cinnamon

Time: 45 minutes| Difficulty: Medium| Serving 2

1 pork tenderloin (about 1 lb.)
2 apples, sliced
1 tsp. cinnamon
1 tbsp. honey
1 tbsp. olive oil
Salt and pepper, to taste

1. Preheat oven to 375°F (190°C).
2. Season pork with salt and pepper.
3. Heat olive oil in a skillet and brown the pork on all sides.
4. Transfer pork to a baking dish, top with apple slices, sprinkle with cinnamon, and drizzle with honey.
5. Roast for 30 minutes or until pork is cooked through.

Per serving
Calories: 295| Protein: 24g| Fat: 14g| Carbs: 18g

Turkey Breast with Apple Stuffing

Time: 1 hour 20 minutes| Difficulty: Medium| Serving 2

1 turkey breast (about 2 lbs.)
2 cups diced apples
1/2 cup diced celery
1 onion, diced
1/4 cup dried cranberries
1 teaspoon dried sage
1 teaspoon dried thyme
Salt and pepper to taste
1 cup low-sodium chicken broth

1. Preheat the oven to 350°F.
2. In a bowl, mix apples, celery, onion, cranberries, sage, and thyme.
3. Season the turkey breast with salt and pepper, and lay flat.
4. Place the stuffing mixture on the turkey, roll up, and tie with kitchen string.
5. Place in a roasting pan and pour chicken broth around the turkey.
6. Roast for about 1 hour or until the internal temperature reaches 165°F.
7. Let rest before slicing.

Per serving: Calories: 290| Protein: 35g| Fat: 6g| Carbs: 22

Pork Tenderloin with Apples and Cinnamon

Time: 45 minutes| Difficulty: Medium| Serving 2

1 pork tenderloin (about 1 lb.)
2 apples, sliced
1 tsp. cinnamon
1 tbsp. honey
1 tbsp. olive oil
Salt and pepper, to taste

6. Preheat oven to 375°F (190°C).
7. Season pork with salt and pepper.
8. Heat olive oil in a skillet and brown the pork on all sides.
9. Transfer pork to a baking dish, top with apple slices, sprinkle with cinnamon, and drizzle with honey.
10. Roast for 30 minutes or until pork is cooked through.

Per serving
Calories: 295| Protein: 24g| Fat: 14g| Carbs: 18g

Turkey Breast with Apple Stuffing

Time: 1 hour 20 minutes| Difficulty: Medium| Serving 2

1 turkey breast (about 2 lbs.)
2 cups diced apples
1/2 cup diced celery
1 onion, diced
1/4 cup dried cranberries
1 teaspoon dried sage
1 teaspoon dried thyme / Salt and pepper to taste
1 cup low-sodium chicken broth

8. Preheat the oven to 350°F.
9. In a bowl, mix apples, celery, onion, cranberries, sage, and thyme.
10. Season the turkey breast with salt and pepper, and lay flat.
11. Place the stuffing mixture on the turkey, roll up, and tie with kitchen string.
12. Place in a roasting pan and pour chicken broth around the turkey.
13. Roast for about 1 hour or until the internal temperature reaches 165°F.
14. Let rest before slicing.

Per serving: Calories: 290| Protein: 35g| Fat: 6g| Carbs: 22

Turkey Meatloaf with Sage and Onion

Time: 1 hour 30 minutes| Difficulty: Easy| Serving 2

1 lb. ground turkey breast
1/2 cup breadcrumbs
1/4 cup milk (use almond milk for lower fat)
1 onion, finely chopped
2 cloves garlic, minced
1 egg, beaten
2 tbsp. fresh sage, chopped and Salt and pepper, to taste

1. Preheat oven to 375°F (190°C).
2. In a bowl, mix all ingredients thoroughly.
3. Shape into a loaf and place in a baking dish.
4. Bake for about 1 hour or until cooked through.

Per serving: Calories: 265| Protein: 28g| Fat: 7g| Carbs: 18g

Herbed Chicken with Roasted Vegetables

Time: 1 hour| Difficulty: Easy| Serving 2

2 boneless, skinless chicken breasts
1 tbsp. olive oil
1 tsp. dried rosemary
1 tsp. dried thyme
Salt and pepper, to taste
1 cup baby carrots
1 cup Brussels sprouts, halved
1 small sweet potato, cubed

1. Preheat oven to 400°F (200°C).
2. Season chicken with olive oil, rosemary, thyme, salt, and pepper.
3. Arrange chicken and vegetables on a baking tray.
4. Roast for 45 minutes, until chicken is cooked through and vegetables are tender.

Per serving: Calories: 310| Protein: 28g| Fat: 14g| Carbs: 22g

Chapter 3: A 28-day Meal Plan for a High-Protein Lifestyle

Week 1: Transition & Getting Acquainted

Day 1:

Breakfast: Greek Yogurt Parfait with Granola and Fruit
Lunch: Turkey and Avocado Wrap with Whole Wheat Tortilla, served with Roasted Brussels Sprouts
Dinner: Lemon Herb Baked Salmon with Quinoa Pilaf and Lemon Garlic Roasted Broccoli

Day 2:

Breakfast: Apple Cinnamon Overnight Oats
Lunch: Tuna Salad Lettuce Wraps, served with Cucumber Avocado Salad
Dinner: Baked Lemon Herb Chicken with Garlic Mashed Cauliflower and Steamed Green Beans.

Day 3:

Breakfast: Broccoli and Cheese Breakfast Casserole
Lunch: Grilled Chicken Salad with Mixed Greens
Dinner: Beef Stir-Fry with Vegetables served with Quinoa Pilaf

Day 4:

Breakfast: Egg and Vegetable Frittata
Lunch: Mediterranean Chickpea Salad
Dinner: Grilled Swordfish with Mango Salsa served with Lemon Herb Quinoa Salad and Grilled Portobello Mushroom Caps

Day 5:

Breakfast: Berry Chia Seed Pudding
Lunch: Black Bean and Corn Salad with Avocado
Dinner: Turkey Chili served with Garlic Herb Roasted Potatoes

Day 6:

Breakfast: Avocado Toast with Poached Eggs
Lunch: Beet and Goat Cheese Salad
Dinner: Chicken Fajitas with Garlic Mashed Cauliflower

Day 7:

Breakfast: Lemon Blueberry Quinoa Breakfast Bowl
Lunch: Quinoa and Black Bean Salad
Dinner: Pork Tenderloin with Apple Compote served with Lemon Garlic Green Beans

Week 2: Introducing Variety

Day 1:

Breakfast: Apple Cinnamon Overnight Oats
Lunch: Turkey and Avocado Wrap with Whole Wheat Tortilla, served with Roasted Brussels Sprouts
Dinner: Lemon Herb Baked Salmon with Quinoa Pilaf and Lemon Garlic Roasted Broccoli

Day 2:

Breakfast: Mango Coconut Chia Pudding
Lunch: Mediterranean Chickpea Salad
Dinner: Beef Stir-Fry with Vegetables served with Quinoa Pilaf

Day 3:

Breakfast: Peanut Butter Banana Toast
Lunch: Greek Salad with Grilled Chicken
Dinner: Grilled Swordfish with Mango Salsa served with Lemon Herb Quinoa Salad and Grilled Portobello Mushroom Caps

Day 4:

Breakfast: Sweet Potato Hash with Turkey Sausage
Lunch: Black Bean and Corn Salad with Avocado
Dinner: Chicken Fajitas with Garlic Mashed Cauliflower

Day 5:

Breakfast: Protein-Packed Breakfast Bowl
Lunch: Caprese Salad with Basil and Balsamic Glaze
Dinner: Turkey Chili served with Garlic Herb Roasted Potatoes

Day 6:

Breakfast: Lemon Blueberry Quinoa Breakfast Bowl
Lunch: Beet and Goat Cheese Salad
Dinner: Pork Tenderloin with Apple Compote served with Lemon Garlic Green Beans

Day 7:

Breakfast: Spinach and Mushroom Omelet
Lunch: Quinoa and Black Bean Salad

Dinner: Grilled Steak with Chimichurri Sauce served with Herb Roasted Potatoes

Week 3: Building Balanced Habits

Day 1:

Breakfast: Greek Yogurt Parfait with Granola and Fruit
Lunch: Turkey and Cranberry Wrap with a Side of Quinoa Pilaf
Dinner: Lemon Herb Baked Salmon with Steamed Asparagus and Lemon Herb Quinoa Salad

Day 2:

Breakfast: Egg Salad Lettuce Wraps
Lunch: Grilled Chicken Salad with Mixed Greens
Dinner: Beef Stir-Fry with Vegetables served with Garlic Mashed Cauliflower

Day 3:

Breakfast: Avocado Toast with Poached Eggs
Lunch: Mediterranean Chickpea Salad
Dinner: Grilled Swordfish with Mango Salsa served with Roasted Brussels Sprouts and Herb Roasted Potatoes

Day 4:

Breakfast: Berry Chia Seed Pudding
Lunch: Tuna Salad Lettuce Wraps with a Side of Quinoa and Black Bean Salad
Dinner: Chicken Fajitas with Quinoa Pilaf and Garlic Roasted Cauliflower

Day 5:

Breakfast: Lemon Blueberry Quinoa Breakfast Bowl
Lunch: Greek Salad with Grilled Chicken
Dinner: Turkey Chili served with Balsamic Glazed Roasted Carrots and Steamed Green Beans with Almonds

Day 6:

Breakfast: Sweet Potato Hash with Turkey Sausage
Lunch: Beet and Goat Cheese Salad
Dinner: Pork Tenderloin with Honey Mustard Glaze served with Lemon Garlic Green Beans and Herb Roasted Potatoes

Day 7:

Breakfast: Spinach and Mushroom Omelet
Lunch: Quinoa and Black Bean Salad

Dinner: Grilled Steak with Chimichurri Sauce served with Grilled Portobello Mushroom Caps and Lemon Herb Quinoa Salad

Week 4: Mastering the High protein Lifestyle

Day 1:

Breakfast: Greek Yogurt Parfait with Granola and Fruit
Lunch: Turkey and Avocado Wrap with Whole Wheat Tortilla, served with Roasted Brussels Sprouts
Dinner: Lemon Herb Baked Salmon with Quinoa Pilaf and Lemon Garlic Roasted Broccoli

Day 2:

Breakfast: Apple Cinnamon Overnight Oats
Lunch: Mediterranean Chickpea Salad
Dinner: Beef Stir-Fry with Vegetables served with Quinoa Pilaf

Day 3:

Breakfast: Avocado Toast with Poached Eggs
Lunch: Grilled Chicken Salad with Mixed Greens
Dinner: Grilled Swordfish with Mango Salsa served with Lemon Herb Quinoa Salad and Grilled Portobello Mushroom Caps

Day 4:

Breakfast: Berry Chia Seed Pudding
Lunch: Black Bean and Corn Salad with Avocado
Dinner: Turkey Chili served with Garlic Herb Roasted Potatoes

Day 5:

Breakfast: Lemon Blueberry Quinoa Breakfast Bowl
Lunch: Greek Salad with Grilled Chicken
Dinner: Pork Tenderloin with Apple Compote served with Lemon Garlic Green Beans and Herb Roasted Potatoes

Day 6:

Breakfast: Sweet Potato Hash with Turkey Sausage
Lunch: Beet and Goat Cheese Salad
Dinner: Chicken Fajitas with Quinoa Pilaf and Garlic Roasted Cauliflower

Day 7:

Breakfast: Spinach and Mushroom Omelet

Chapter 6: Washing and Handling

The importance of proper cleaning

Before getting into the complexities of plant-based cuisine, it's critical to grasp the significance of carefully cleaning fruits and vegetables. This removes dirt, bacteria, and pesticide residues, making your dishes both delicious and safe.

Step-by-Step Guide to Washing Produce:

1. Hand Hygiene: Wash hands thoroughly with warm water and soap before and after preparing fruits and vegetables. This critical step reduces the spread of microorganisms to your food.

2. Make a Vinegar and Salt Solution: In a large dish, combine 1 1/3 cups vinegar and 1 tablespoon salt. Stir the mixture until the vinegar and salt are completely dissolved. Rest certain that the vinegar, a natural disinfectant, and the salt, a microbe-drawing aid, will work together to thoroughly clean your vegetables.

3. Initial Rinse: Wash fruits and vegetables under running water. Gently rub the surface to remove dirt and insecticides. Avoid using soap or chemical cleansers, as these might leave toxic residues if consumed.

4. Soaking times vary depending on the sort of product. Thin-skinned fruits and vegetables, such as berries and leafy greens, require only a 5-minute soak in the vinegar and salt solution. Firm-skinned food, such as apples and squash, should be left in the solution for 10 minutes. This step is crucial to complete disinfection.

5. Scrubbing: Using a clean vegetable brush, gently scrub the skins of complex and textured fruits and vegetables such as melons, carrots, sweet potatoes, and cucumbers. This eliminates trapped dirt and bacteria that a simple rinse may not have removed.

6. Rinsing Post-Soak: After soaking and washing, rinse the vegetables with plain water to eliminate any remaining vinegar or salt. Rinse well to remove any remaining remains.

7. Drying: To dry the fruits and veggies, use a clean kitchen cloth or paper towel. This step is not simply for convenience; it also reduces the possibility of bacterial growth.

8. Inspect and Cut: Check your vegetables for damaged or bruised regions. Cut these away since they can harbor bacteria and degrade the quality and safety of your meal.
Use separate chopping boards for fruits, vegetables, and uncooked meat. After each use, thoroughly clean the board with hot, soapy water.

9. Meat: To avoid cross-contamination, wash your hands, meat, and utensils with soap and hot water, and then pat dry before seasoning or cooking. Follow the right cooking temperatures and times to ensure the meat is safely prepared and cooked to the recommended internal temperature.

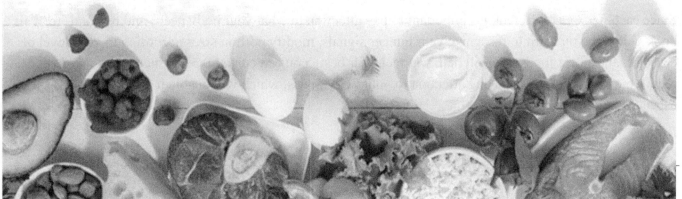

Conclusion

By the time you finish reading "Low-Carb High-Protein Cookbook for Beginners," I hope you'll be more prepared, motivated, and eager to keep cooking. This book has been thoughtfully written to act as a thorough guide, supporting you in adopting a nourishing lifestyle that places an emphasis on high-quality protein and reduces needless carbs.

Making the switch to a high-protein, low-carb diet is a commitment to enhance your general health and wellbeing, not merely a food adjustment. You can gain a variety of benefits by concentrating on nutrient-dense foods, such as improved energy and metabolic health, weight control, and muscular growth. This eating style can change your connection with food and your body, resulting in a more balanced and conscious way of living.

We've looked at a wide range of delectable recipes in this cookbook that suit various palates, dietary requirements, and events. Every meal, from filling dinners to robust breakfasts, is created to be both tasty and nourishing, so you never have to give up flavor for health. The goal of including useful advice and techniques is to facilitate your transition and provide you the means to sustain this way of life in the long run.

THINKING BACK ON THE MAIN IDEAS

KNOWLEDGE BASED EMPOWERMENT
Any successful diet change starts with knowledge. Knowing the fundamentals of a high-protein, low-carb diet gives you the power to make wise decisions. This cookbook has given you a clear road map for everything from knowing what basic ingredients and kitchen tools are to learning how to organize and create healthy meals. You can more confidently handle your food path if you take this advice to heart.

THE VALUE OF BEING READY

The secret to maintaining any lifestyle change is preparation. This book's recipes and meal plans highlight the value of prepping ahead of time, cooking in large quantities, and maintaining a well-stocked kitchen. You may steer clear of the dangers of convenience meals and make sure that wholesome, fulfilling options are available by setting aside time to prepare.

PAYING ATTENTION TO YOUR BODY

Since each person is different, it's important to pay attention to what your body needs and responds to. This book will help you learn to recognize your hunger signals, modify portion sizes according to your level of exercise, and select foods that will help you feel your best. You can customize this diet to fit your unique requirements and tastes by paying attention to your body's cues, which will enable it to become a long-term aspect of your lifestyle.

BUILDING A SUPPORT SYSTEM

Starting a diet adjustment is simpler with support. It might be as simple as sharing your journey with friends and family or as complex as consulting nutritionists, but having a support system can help with accountability and inspiration. This book urges you to create and use your support system to stay on course and recognize your accomplishments.

LOOKING AHEAD

As you delve deeper into high-protein, low-carb eating, remember that balance and consistency are crucial. It's critical to have an open mind and to keep trying new things to discover new ingredients and recipes that will add excitement and enjoyment to your meals. Your adventure will continue as you develop and adjust to your shifting dietary requirements and tastes.

Think of extending your culinary horizons in the future by experimenting with new recipes, learning intricate techniques, or even cultivating your own fresh vegetables. You've only just begun to use the abilities and information this cookbook has given you. Use them as a starting point to create a lifetime of delectable, healthful food. Let the joy of culinary exploration fill your kitchen with excitement and adventure.

LAST WORDS

More than just a cookbook, "Low-Carb High-Protein Cookbook for Beginners" celebrates a more energetic, healthful way of life. You're investing wisely in your future well-being and happiness when you choose this lifestyle. I hope this book has ignited a passion for wholesome, flavorful cuisine that will only develop. Cooking should be a joyous, creative activity. Let the celebration of a healthful lifestyle inspire and motivate you.

I am grateful that you let me share in your adventure. May the smells of home-cooked meals fill your kitchen, and may your table be a source of happiness and sustenance.

Cheers to a happy and healthier you

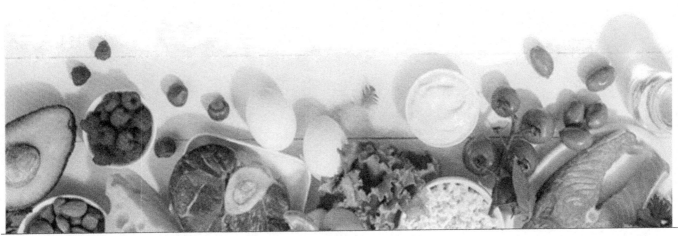

Made in the USA
Monee, IL
17 November 2024

70412904R00059